BARIATRIC COOKBOOK

DINNER BUNDLE

GASTRIC BYPASS COOKBOOK: MAIN COURSE

70+ Bariatric-Friendly Chicken, Beef, Fish, Pork, Fish, Salads
and Vegetarian recipes for lifelong eating
for Post Weight Loss Surgery Diet

GASTRIC BYPASS COOKBOOK: SLOW COOKER

50+ Bariatric-Friendly Chicken, Beef, Pork and Vegetarian
Slow Cooker Recipes for Life Long Eating
for Post Weight Loss Surgery Diet

STELLA LAYNE

GASTRIC BYPASS COOKBOOK: MAIN COURSE

GASTRIC BYPASS COOKBOOK: SLOW COOKER

BEEF RECIPES

CHICKEN RECIPES

PORK RECIPES

VEGETARIAN RECIPES

COOKING INFO SUMMARY

NUTRITION SUMMARY

BEEF AND VEGETABLES STIR FRY

 SERVES **8**

 PREP TIME **15** MINUTES

 COOK TIME **10** MINUTES

- **1 pound** lean flank steak, cut into strips

- **1/4 cup** fat-free beef broth

- **2 cups** broccoli florets

- **1 cup** sliced bell peppers

- **1 cup** sliced carrot

- **1** green onion, chopped

- **2 cloves** garlic, minced

- **2 tablespoons** low sodium soy sauce

- **1 tablespoon** grated ginger

- **1 teaspoon** stevia

1. In a small bowl, mix beef with soy sauce, stevia and ginger. Set aside to marinate for 10 minutes.

2. Spray a large skillet. Sauté the onion until fragrant. Then add all the vegetables. Cook for 4-5 minutes until vegetables are tender. Remove from the skillet.

3. Add the beef. Reserve the marinade. Cook until the beef is brown. Then return the vegetables, broth and marinade. Stir and cook for 2 minutes.

CALORIES	CARBS	SUGAR	FAT	PROTEIN	SODIUM
99	4.6	1.9	2.6	13.4	337
KCAL	GRAMS	GRAMS	GRAMS	GRAMS	MILLIGRAMS

THAI GROUND BEEF

 SERVES 8

 PREP TIME 10 MINUTES

 COOK TIME 20 MINUTES

1. Spray a large skillet.

2. Sauté the leek until fragrant. Then add garlic and sauté for 1 more minute.

3. Brown the beef.

4. Stir in curry paste and tomato sauce. Simmer for 3-4 minutes or until the liquid is reduced to half.

5. Stir in the coconut milk and seasoning. Bring to a boil. Serve immediately.

- **1 pound** 95/5 lean ground beef
- **2 cloves** garlic, minced
- **1 cup** thinly sliced leek
- **1 cup** no-sugar-added tomato sauce
- **1/2 cup** light coconut milk
- **1 tablespoon** red curry paste
- **1/2 tablespoon** stevia
- **1/2 tablespoon** fish sauce
- **1/2 tablespoon** lime juice
- **1/2 teaspoon** Sriracha sauce (optional)
- **1/4 teaspoon** lime zest
- salt and pepper to taste
- Nonstick Cooking Spray

CALORIES	CARBS	SUGAR	FAT	PROTEIN	SODIUM
106	4.1	2.1	3.9	13.0	270
KCAL	GRAMS	GRAMS	GRAMS	GRAMS	MILLIGRAMS

SPICY BEEF WITH BOK CHOY

 SERVES
8

 PREP TIME
15
MINUTES

 COOK TIME
20
MINUTES

- **1 pound** lean flank steak, cut into strips

- **6 heads** baby Bok Choy, cut in half

- **1 cup** sliced onion

- **2 cloves** garlic, minced

- **2** chili peppers, deseeded and chopped

- **1 tablespoon** grated ginger

- 2 tablespoons fish sauce

- 1/4 teaspoon salt

- 1/4 teaspoon pepper

- Nonstick Cooking Spray

1. In a medium bowl, season the beef with salt and pepper.

2. Sauté the garlic, ginger and chili until fragrant. Add the beef and cook for 3 minutes. Set Aside.

3. Sauté the onion until fragrant.

4. Then add Bok Choy and cook until soft.

5. Add the beef and fish sauce. Mix well and cook for 1 minute.

CALORIES	CARBS	SUGAR	FAT	PROTEIN	SODIUM
114	5.7	1.6	2.6	13.5	469
KCAL	GRAMS	GRAMS	GRAMS	GRAMS	MILLIGRAMS

BEEF STUFFED BELL PEPPER

 SERVES
8

 PREP TIME
5
MINUTES

 COOK TIME
35
MINUTES

1. Preheat the oven to 375°F.

2. Spray a large skillet.

3. Sauté the onion until fragrant. Then add garlic, green onion

4. and green peppers. Sauté for 3 more minutes. Set aside.

5. Brown the beef. Then all ingredients except cheese and tomato sauce. Mix well and cook for another 5 minutes.

6. Fill the bell peppers half the way with the meat mixture. Add cheddar cheese. Then add the remaining meat mixture. Top with tomato sauce and mozzarella cheese.

7. Bake for 20-25 minutes.

- **1 pound** 95/5 lean ground beef
- **4 medium** green bell peppers, tops and seeds removed
- **1 cup** canned diced tomatoes
- **1/3 cup** finely chopped onion
- **1/4 cup** finely chopped green onion
- **1/4 cup** fat-free mozzarella cheese
- **1/4 cup** fat-free cheddar cheese
- **1/2 cup** no-sugar-added tomato and pesto sauce
- **2 cloves** garlic, minced
- **2 tablespoons** minced green peppers
- **2 tablespoons** chopped fresh parsley
- **1 1/2 teaspoons** Italian seasoning
- 1 teaspoon salt
- **1/2 teaspoon** ground black pepper
- Nonstick Cooking Spray

CALORIES	CARBS	SUGAR	FAT	PROTEIN	SODIUM
118	7.7	3.6	3.2	15.6	471
KCAL	GRAMS	GRAMS	GRAMS	GRAMS	MILLIGRAMS

SALISBURY STEAK WITH MUSHROOM SAUCE

SERVES
8

PREP TIME
15
MINUTES

COOK TIME
25
MINUTES

For the Salisbury Steak

- **1 pound** 95/5 lean ground beef
- **1/4 cup** whole wheat bread crumbs
- **1/4 cup** chopped onion
- **2** egg whites, beaten
- **1 teaspoon** salt
- Nonstick Cooking Spray

For the Gravy

- **2 cups** fat-free beef broth
- **1 1/2 cups** sliced onion
- **1 cup** sliced mushrooms
- **2 tablespoons** whole wheat flour
- salt and pepper to taste

1. Combine all ingredients for the steak. Shape into 8 mini patties.

2. Spray a large skillet. Brown the Steak on both sides over medium heat, about 4-5 minutes each side.

3. Add broth, onion and mushroom. Bring to a boil then reduce to low. Cover and simmer for 10 more minutes. Transfer the patties to the serving plate.

4. In a small bowl, combine flour with a few tablespoons of water. Then slowly stir in the mixture. Cook until sauce thickened. Pour the sauce on the steak and serve.

CALORIES	CARBS	SUGAR	FAT	PROTEIN	SODIUM
120	50	0.9	2.9	17.0	566
KCAL	GRAMS	GRAMS	GRAMS	GRAMS	MILLIGRAMS

MEXICAN BEEF SKILLET

SERVES
8

PREP TIME
10
MINUTES

COOK TIME
35
MINUTES

1. In a medium bowl, season the beef with chili powder, salt and paprika.

2. Spray a large skillet, cook the beef for 3 minutes. Set aside.

3. Sauté the garlic, onion and bell peppers until fragrant. Then add mushroom and cook for another 2 minutes.

4. Add broth and salsa. Simmer until the liquid is reduced by half. Stir in beef and cook for 1 minute.

- **1 pound** lean flank steak, cut into strips

- **1 cup** sliced onion

- **1 cup** sliced mushroom

- **1 cup** sliced red bell pepper

- **3/4 cup** fat-free low sodium chicken broth

- **1/2 cup** no-sugar-added salsa

- **2 cloves** garlic, minced

- **2 teaspoons** chili powder

- 1 teaspoon paprika

- 1/2 teaspoon salt

- Nonstick Cooking Spray

CALORIES	CARBS	SUGAR	FAT	PROTEIN	SODIUM
102	4.4	1.9	2.7	13.2	339
KCAL	GRAMS	GRAMS	GRAMS	GRAMS	MILLIGRAMS

INDIAN BEEF CURRY

 SERVES
8

 PREP TIME
10
MINUTES

 COOK TIME
40
MINUTES

- **1 pound** 95/5 lean ground beef

- **1** 14.5-ounce **can** diced tomatoes

- **1 cup** chopped onion

- **1/2 cup** frozen peas, thawed

- **1 cup** fat-free beef broth

- **1/2 cup** fat-free Greek Yogurt

- **2 cloves** garlic, minced

- **2 tablespoons** curry powder

- **1/2 teaspoon** chili paste

- **1/4 teaspoon** ground turmeric

- salt to taste

- **2 tablespoons** chopped fresh Parsley

1. Spray a large skillet.

2. Sauté the onion until fragrant. Then add garlic and sauté for 1 more minute.

3. Brown the beef. Transfer the beef mixture to a bowl.

4. Add turmeric, curry powder and chili paste. Cook for 30 seconds.

5. Slowly stir in broth and tomatoes. Add Peas. Bring to a boil. Simmer for 15 minutes or until the peas soften.

6. Add beef mixture back. Season with salt.

7. Remove from heat. Stir in yogurt and sprinkle with chopped parsley.

CALORIES	CARBS	SUGAR	FAT	PROTEIN	SODIUM
113	6.4	2.9	3.3	15.0	316
KCAL	GRAMS	GRAMS	GRAMS	GRAMS	MILLIGRAMS

SKINNY ENCHILADAS

 SERVES
9

 PREP TIME
10
MINUTES

 COOK TIME
45
MINUTES

1. Preheat the oven to 350°F

2. Spray a large skillet.

3. Sauté the onion until fragrant. Then Brown the beef. Season with salt and pepper.

4. In a large bowl, combine yogurt, soup and half of the cheese.

5. Mix half of the soup mixture with the meat. Divide the meat between tortillas. Roll up and place them in a baking dish. Top with the remaining sauce and cheese.

6. Bake for 30 minutes.

- **1 pound** 95/5 lean ground beef
- **3** low carb tortillas
- **1** 10.5-ounce **can** condensed 98% fat-free cream of chicken soup
- **1/2 cup** chopped green onions
- **1/2 cup** fat-free Greek yogurt
- **1 1/2 cups** fat-free mozzarella cheese
- **1** jalapeno pepper, de-seeded and chopped
- **2 tablespoons** Taco seasoning
- salt and pepper to taste

CALORIES	CARBS	SUGAR	FAT	PROTEIN	SODIUM
149	7.5	0.6	4.3	19.9	495
KCAL	GRAMS	GRAMS	GRAMS	GRAMS	MILLIGRAMS

BEEF CHILI

 SERVES
8

 PREP TIME
10
MINUTES

 COOK TIME
60
MINUTES

- **1 pound** 95/5 lean ground beef

- **1** 15-ounce **can** dark red kidney beans, rinsed and drained

- **1/2 cup** chopped onion

- **1 1/2 cups** no-sugar-added tomato juice

- **1/2 cup** no-sugar-added salsa

- **1 tablespoon** chili powder

- **1/2 tablespoon** garlic powder

- **1/2 teaspoon** ground cumin

- **1/2 teaspoon** paprika

- **1/4 teaspoon** thyme

1. Spray a large skillet.

2. Sauté the onion until fragrant. Then Brown the beef.

3. Add all ingredients and mix well. Bring to a boil. Reduce to low and simmer for 50 minutes. Season with salt and pepper.

CALORIES	CARBS	SUGAR	FAT	PROTEIN	SODIUM
147	14.6	3.7	3.3	15.7	227
KCAL	GRAMS	GRAMS	GRAMS	GRAMS	MILLIGRAMS

CHEESE-STUFFED MEATLOAF

SERVES
8

PREP TIME
20
MINUTES

COOK TIME
60
MINUTES

1. Preheat the oven to 350°F

2. In a large mixing bowl, combine all ingredients except cheese.

3. Spread the meat mixture on a large baking sheet to form a 14"x18" patty.

4. Add the cheese on the meat. Leave out 1-inch on each side.

5. Roll up and Put it in a 10"x15" baking dish.

6. Bake for 1 hour.

- **2 pounds** 95/5 lean ground beef

- **1/2 cup** whole wheat breadcrumbs

- **1/2 cup** chopped onion

- **4** egg whites, beaten

- **2 cups** fat-free shredded cheddar cheese

- **1 1/2 teaspoons** salt

- **1 1/2 teaspoons** ground black pepper

CALORIES	CARBS	SUGAR	FAT	PROTEIN	SODIUM
83	3.6	0.5	1.6	13.7	412
KCAL	GRAMS	GRAMS	GRAMS	GRAMS	MILLIGRAMS

ITALIAN PARMESAN MEATBALLS

 SERVES **8**

 PREP TIME **20** MINUTES

 COOK TIME **70** MINUTES

- **1 pound** 95/5 lean ground beef
- **1/4 cup** whole wheat breadcrumbs
- **1/4 cup** fat-free shredded Parmesan Cheese
- **1/4 cup** fat-free shredded mozzarella cheese
- **1 1/4 cups** No-sugar-added tomato and basil sauce
- **1 1/2 tablespoons** Italian Seasoning
- **1/2 teaspoon** salt
- **1/2 teaspoon** ground black pepper
- **2 tablespoons** chopped fresh parsley

1. Preheat the oven to 350°F

2. In a large mixing bowl, combine beef, breadcrumbs, parmesan cheese, 1/4 cup of the tomato sauce and seasoning. Shape into 8 meatballs.

3. Bake for 15 minutes.

4. On an oven-proof skillet, add the remaining sauce and the meatballs. Toss well. Top with the mozzarella cheese and bake to another 15 minutes. Sprinkle with parsley before serving.

CALORIES	CARBS	SUGAR	FAT	PROTEIN	SODIUM
116	6.7	1.9	3.4	14.7	454
KCAL	GRAMS	GRAMS	GRAMS	GRAMS	MILLIGRAMS

CABBAGE AND BEEF BAKE

SERVES
12

PREP TIME
15
MINUTES

COOK TIME
80
MINUTES

1. Preheat the oven to 350°F

2. Spray a large skillet.

3. Sauté the onion and bell peppers until fragrant. Then Brown the beef. Stir in Tomatoes. Season with salt and pepper Set aside.

4. Spray a 9"x13" baking dish. Spread the shredded cabbage evenly. Then spread the meat mixture on top.

5. In a small bowl, mix together tomato sauce and sour cream. Then spread the mixture on the meat.

6. Bake for 1 hour. Then top with cheese and bake for another 20 minutes.

- **1 1/2 pounds** 95/5 lean ground beef

- **6 cups** shredded cabbage

- **1 cup** chopped onion

- **1/2 cup** chopped bell peppers

- 1 14.5-ounce **can** diced tomato

- 1 8-ounce **can** tomato sauce

- **1 cup** fat-free sour cream

- **1/2 cup** fat-free shredded cheddar cheese

- **1/2 cup** fat-free shredded mozzarella cheese

- salt and pepper to taste

CALORIES	CARBS	SUGAR	FAT	PROTEIN	SODIUM
131	9.0	4.8	3.1	17.6	313
KCAL	GRAMS	GRAMS	GRAMS	GRAMS	MILLIGRAMS

BEER BRAISED BEEF

 SERVES
16

 PREP TIME
5
MINUTES

 COOK TIME
3
HOURS

- **2 pounds** lean top round roast
- **2 cans** beer
- **2** large onion, sliced
- **4 cloves** garlic
- **1 teaspoon** salt
- **1 teaspoon** Ground Thyme
- **1/2 teaspoon** Rosemary
- **1/2 teaspoon** ground black pepper
- Nonstick cooking spray

1. Preheat the oven to 275°F

2. Spray a large Dutch oven. Sauté the onion until fragrant. Set aside.

3. Season the meat with salt and pepper. Brown the meat on all side for about 2 minutes per side. Add all ingredients.

4. Cover and cook in the oven for 2 3/4 to 3 hours.

5. Shred the meat with a pair of forks before serving.

CALORIES	CARBS	SUGAR	FAT	PROTEIN	SODIUM
96	3.6	0.8	2.0	13.0	247
KCAL	GRAMS	GRAMS	GRAMS	GRAMS	MILLIGRAMS

SICHUAN SPICY BEEF STEW

 SERVES 16

 PREP TIME 15 MINUTES

 COOK TIME 2 HOURS

1. Blanch the beef in boiling water. Drain and set aside.

2. Spray a wok. Sauté the ginger and garlic until fragrant. Add the chili paste and cook for 30 seconds.

3. Add beef, soy sauce and wine. Stir well and cook for 2 minutes.

4. Transfer to a stock pot. Add the spices and enough water to cover the beef. Bring to a boil and reduce to low. Simmer for 1 hour.

5. Add Radish. Cook for another 30 minutes or until both beef and radish are tender. Garnish with cilantro and serve.

- **2 pounds** lean top round roast, cut into 1 1/2 slices across the grain
- **1 pound** radish, cut into 2-inch pieces
- **5 cloves** garlic, minced
- **4 slices** fresh ginger
- **3 tablespoons** dry white wine
- **2 tablespoons** chopped fresh cilantro
- **1 tablespoon** Sichuan chilli bean paste
- **1 tablespoon** low-sodium soy sauce
- Nonstick Cooking Spray

Spices:

- **4** dried chili
- **2** star anise
- **2** bay leaves
- **1** cinnamon stick
- **1 teaspoon** peppercorn
- **1 teaspoon** fennel seeds

CALORIES	CARBS	SUGAR	FAT	PROTEIN	SODIUM
84	2.4	0.7	2.0	13.0	102
KCAL	GRAMS	GRAMS	GRAMS	GRAMS	MILLIGRAMS

MONGOLIAN BEEF SKEWER

SERVES
8

PREP TIME
8
HOURS

COOK TIME
10
MINUTES

- **1 pound** lean flank steak, cut into strips

- **2 tablespoons** low-sodium soy sauce

- **2 tablespoons** sherry cooking wine

- **1 tablespoon** grated ginger

- **1 tablespoon** minced garlic

- **2 teaspoons** Truvia Nectar

- **1 teaspoon** dried mustard powder

1. In a large resealable bag, add all ingredients. Seal and shake the bag to mix well. Marinate overnight.

2. Preheat the broiler. Thread the meat onto 16 skewers.

3. Broil 3-4 minutes on each side.

CALORIES	CARBS	SUGAR	FAT	PROTEIN	SODIUM
90	1.8	1.0	2.6	12.3	210
KCAL	GRAMS	GRAMS	GRAMS	GRAMS	MILLIGRAMS

CHICKEN AND SUGAR SNAP PEA STIR FRY

 SERVES 8

 PREP TIME 10 MINUTES

 COOK TIME 15 MINUTES

1. Spray a large skillet. Brown the chicken. Add oyster sauce and cook for another minute. Set aside.

2. Sauté green onion and garlic until fragrant. Then add peas and cook until fragrant. Stir in chicken and stir-fry for 30 seconds.

- **1 pound** chicken tender, cut into strips
- **12 ounces** sugar snap peas, , cut into strips
- **1 tablespoon** oyster sauce
- **2 cloves** garlic, minced
- **2** green onions, chopped
- salt and pepper to taste

CALORIES	CARBS	SUGAR	FAT	PROTEIN	SODIUM
59	1.7	0.6	0.3	11.5	118
KCAL	GRAMS	GRAMS	GRAMS	GRAMS	MILLIGRAMS

LEMON THYME CHICKEN

 SERVES
8

 PREP TIME
15
MINUTES

 COOK TIME
20
MINUTES

- **1 pound** chicken tender

- **1/4 cup** lemon juice

- **6 sprigs** fresh thyme, chopped

- **1 tablespoon** lemon zest

- **2 cloves** garlic, minced

- salt and pepper to taste

- Nonstick Cooking Spray

1. In a large bowl, mix the chicken in all other ingredients. Set aside to marinate for 15 minutes.

2. Spray a large skillet. Cook the chicken until cook through, about 4-5 minutes each side

CALORIES	CARBS	SUGAR	FAT	PROTEIN	SODIUM
55	1.0	0.2	0.2	11.3	56
KCAL	GRAMS	GRAMS	GRAMS	GRAMS	MILLIGRAMS

PEPPER-STUFFED CAJUN CHICKEN

 SERVES
8

 PREP TIME
10
MINUTES

 COOK TIME
25
MINUTES

1. Preheat the oven to 350°F.

2. Spray a large skillet.

3. Sauté the onion and bell peppers until fragrant. Season with salt and pepper. Set aside to cool.

4. Slice the chicken breast to form a pocket. Stuff the vegetable and then the cheese.

5. Rub the Cajun seasoning, then salt and pepper on all side of the chicken breast.

6. Bake for 25 minutes

- **4** boneless, skinless chicken breast

- **1 cup** chopped onion

- **1 cup** chopped bell peppers

- **1 cup** fat free cheddar cheese

- **1 tablespoon** Cajun seasoning

- salt and pepper to taste

- Nonstick Cooking Spray

CALORIES	CARBS	SUGAR	FAT	PROTEIN	SODIUM
91	4.0	1.6	0.6	16.3	522
KCAL	GRAMS	GRAMS	GRAMS	GRAMS	MILLIGRAMS

SPINACH FETA CHICKEN ROLL

 SERVES **8**

 PREP TIME **10** MINUTES

 COOK TIME **25** MINUTES

- **4** boneless, skinless chicken breast, flattened

- **10 ounces** frozen spinach, thawed and squeeze

- **1/2 cup** fat-free feta cheese

- **1/3 cup** fat-free ricotta cheese

- **1/4 cup** chopped green onion

- **1/4 cup** chopped fresh parsley

- **1 tablespoon** fresh dill

- **2 cloves** garlic

- salt and pepper to taste

1. Preheat the oven to 350°F.

2. Spray a large skillet.

3. Sauté the green onion and garlic until fragrant. Add spinach, parsley and dill. Cool until heated through. Season with salt and pepper.

4. Remove from heat and stir in feta cheese and ricotta cheese.

5. Divide the mixture onto the chicken breast. Roll up. Rub the chicken with salt and pepper.

6. Bake for 25 minutes.

CALORIES	CARBS	SUGAR	FAT	PROTEIN	SODIUM
83	2.1	0.8	0.6	15.0	328
KCAL	GRAMS	GRAMS	GRAMS	GRAMS	MILLIGRAMS

CREAMY SALSA CHICKEN

 SERVES
8

 PREP TIME
5
MINUTES

 COOK TIME
35
MINUTES

1. Preheat the oven to 350°F.

2. Season the chicken with half of the taco seasoning.

3. Brown the chicken in an -oven-proof skillet. Then stir in salsa and the remaining seasoning.

4. Cover and bake for 30 minutes.

5. Shred the chicken and stir in sour cream.

- **1 pound** chicken tender

- **2 cups** salsa

- **1 package** taco seasoning

- **1 cup** fat-free soup cream

- Nonstick Cooking Spray

CALORIES	CARBS	SUGAR	FAT	PROTEIN	SODIUM
92	5.5	4.0	0.2	12.0	296
KCAL	GRAMS	GRAMS	GRAMS	GRAMS	MILLIGRAMS

YOGURT CHICKEN PARMESAN

 SERVES
8

 PREP TIME
10
MINUTES

 COOK TIME
45
MINUTES

- **1 pound** chicken tender

- **1/2 cup** fat-free Greek Yogurt

- **1/2 cup** low-fat mayonnaise

- **1/2 cup** fat-free grated parmesan cheese

- **1/2 teaspoon** salt

- **1/2 teaspoon** ground black pepper

1. Preheat the oven to 375°F.

2. In a medium bowl, mix yogurt, mayonnaise, cheese and seasonings.

3. Line the chicken on a baking tray. Spread the mixture on the chicken breast.

4. Bake for 45 minutes.

CALORIES	CARBS	SUGAR	FAT	PROTEIN	SODIUM
88	5.6	1.4	1.2	13.4	463
KCAL	GRAMS	GRAMS	GRAMS	GRAMS	MILLIGRAMS

HUNGARIAN CHICKEN PAPRIKASH

SERVES
8

PREP TIME
10
MINUTES

COOK TIME
50
MINUTES

1. Season the chicken with salt and pepper. Spray a large skillet. Brown the chicken. Set aside.

2. Sauté the onion until fragrant. Add paprika and cook for 2 minutes. Add broth, tomato and chicken. Bring to a boil then reduce to low. Cover and simmer for 30 minutes.

3. Remove from heat and stir in sour cream before serving.

- **1 pound** chicken tender

- **1 cup** chopped onion

- **2** plum tomatoes, cubed

- **1 cup** fat-free low sodium chicken broth

- **1/4 cup** fat free sour cream

- **1 tablespoon** sweet paprika

- **1 teaspoon** smoked paprika

- salt and pepper to taste

CALORIES	CARBS	SUGAR	FAT	PROTEIN	SODIUM
72	3.7	1.9	0.4	12.2	80
KCAL	GRAMS	GRAMS	GRAMS	GRAMS	MILLIGRAMS

ROSEMARY BRAISED CHICKEN

 SERVES
8

 PREP TIME
5
MINUTES

 COOK TIME
55
MINUTES

- **1 pound** chicken tender

- **1 cup** white wine

- **3 sprigs** fresh rosemary

- **2** bay leave

- **1** lemon, juice only

- salt and pepper to taste

1. Preheat the oven to 375°F.

2. Season the chicken with salt and pepper.

3. In an oven-proof skillet, Brown the chicken. Add wine and herbs. Cook until the sauce reduces by half. Then add 1 1/2 cups water and bring to a boil.

4. Cover and bake for 45 minutes. Stir in lemon juice before serving.

CALORIES	CARBS	SUGAR	FAT	PROTEIN	SODIUM
81	1.2	0.5	0.3	11.0	57
KCAL	GRAMS	GRAMS	GRAMS	GRAMS	MILLIGRAMS

INDONESIAN COCONUT CHICKEN OPOR

SERVES
8

PREP TIME
5
MINUTES

COOK TIME
60
MINUTES

1. Blend all ingredients for the opor paste except lemongrass until smooth.

2. Brown the chicken. Then Brown the Tofu. Set aside.

3. Sauté the paste for 1 minute. Then add all ingredients except coconut milk. Add 4 cups of water. Bring to a boil then reduce to low. Cover and simmer for 45 minutes or until chicken is tender.

4. Stir in coconut milk and simmer, uncovered, for another 10 minutes.

Main Ingredients

- 1 pound chicken tender
- 10 ounce firm tofu, cut into bite-size pieces
- 1 1/2 cups light coconut milk
- 1/2 cups low sodium chicken broth
- Nonstick Cooking Spray

Opor Paste

- 10 shallots
- 10 cloves garlic
- 3 fresh bay leaves
- 2 lemongrass
- 1 tablespoon freshly grated ginger
- 2 teaspoons coriander powder
- 1 teaspoon ground turmeric
- 1/2 teaspoon salt
- 1/4 teaspoon pepper

CALORIES	CARBS	SUGAR	FAT	PROTEIN	SODIUM
136	9.0	1.1	4.1	15.5	226
KCAL	GRAMS	GRAMS	GRAMS	GRAMS	MILLIGRAMS

ITALIAN STUFFED CHICKEN BREAST

SERVES
8

PREP TIME
20
MINUTES

COOK TIME
45
MINUTES

- **4** boneless, skinless chicken breasts, pounded

- **2** plum tomatoes, diced

- **2** red peppers, chopped

- **1 1/2 cups** marinara sauce

- **1 cup** fat-free shredded mozzarella cheese

- **2 tablespoons** chopped fresh basil

- **1 1/2 tablespoons** chopped fresh oregano

- salt and pepper to taste

1. Preheat the oven to 375°F.

2. Season the chicken with salt and pepper.

3. Cook tomatoes, peppers and herbs until hot. Remove from heat and stir in half the cheese. Season with salt and pepper.

4. Divide the mixture onto each chicken breast. Roll up and put in a baking dish.

5. Spread the marinara sauce on the chicken then top with the remaining cheese. Bake for 45 minutes.

CALORIES	CARBS	SUGAR	FAT	PROTEIN	SODIUM
104	5.5	1.7	1.0	16.9	327
KCAL	GRAMS	GRAMS	GRAMS	GRAMS	MILLIGRAMS

WHITE BEAN AND CHICKEN CHILI

 SERVES 8

 PREP TIME 40 MINUTES

 COOK TIME 25 MINUTES

1. Season the chicken with salt and pepper. Spray a large skillet. Brown the chicken. Set aside.

2. Sauté onion until fragrant. Add garlic, chili, cumin, coriander and chili powder. Cook for 1 minute. Add chicken and broth back to the pot. Cover and simmer for 30 minutes.

3. Remove the chicken and add the white beans. Shred the chicken and return to the pot. Simmer for 5-10 minutes until the sauce reduces to desired consistency.

- **1 pound** chicken tender
- 1 15.5-ounce **can** white beans, rinsed and drained
- **2 ounces** diced green chilies
- **1 cup** chopped onion
- 1 poblano chili, seeded and chopped
- **2 cloves** garlic, minced
- **2 cups** low sodium chicken broth
- **1 teaspoon** chili powder
- **1 teaspoon** ground cumin
- **1 teaspoon** ground coriander
- salt and pepper to taste

CALORIES	CARBS	SUGAR	FAT	PROTEIN	SODIUM
115	12.0	1.7	0.6	15.2	322
KCAL	GRAMS	GRAMS	GRAMS	GRAMS	MILLIGRAMS

NORTHERN ITALIAN CHICKEN STEW

 SERVES
8

 PREP TIME
10
MINUTES

 COOK TIME
60
MINUTES

- **1 pound** chicken tender

- **1/2 cup** chopped onion

- **1/2 cup** sliced carrot

- **1/2 cup** sliced red bell pepper

- **1 cup** crushed tomatoes

- **2 cloves** garlic, minced

- **1** bay leave

- **2 tablespoons** dry white wine

- **1 tablespoon** chopped fresh parsley

- **1 teaspoon** minced rosemary

1. Season the chicken with salt and pepper. Spray a large skillet. Brown the chicken. Set aside.

2. Sauté the onion, carrot, bell peppers, garlic, bay leave and rosemary until fragrant. Add wine, tomato and chicken. Bring to a boil then reduce to low. Cover and simmer for 30 minutes.

CALORIES	CARBS	SUGAR	FAT	PROTEIN	SODIUM
77	4.8	2.4	0.3	11.9	145
KCAL	GRAMS	GRAMS	GRAMS	GRAMS	MILLIGRAMS

MUSTARD AND WINE BRAISED CHICKEN

 SERVES
8

 PREP TIME
10
MINUTES

 COOK TIME
60
MINUTES

1. Preheat the oven to 375°F.

2. Season the chicken with salt and pepper. Spray a large skillet. Brown the chicken. Set aside.

3. Sauté onion, garlic and shallots until fragrant. Add chicken, wine, mustard and broth back to the pot. Cover and bake for 45 minutes.

- **1 pound** chicken tender
- **2** shallots, chopped
- **2 cloves** garlic, minced
- **3/4 cup** low sodium chicken broth
- **1/2 cup** dry white wine
- **2 tablespoons** mustard
- **1 tablespoon** chopped fresh thyme
- salt and pepper to taste

CALORIES	CARBS	SUGAR	FAT	PROTEIN	SODIUM
71	1.6	0.6	0.3	11.4	105
KCAL	GRAMS	GRAMS	GRAMS	GRAMS	MILLIGRAMS

YAKITORI CHICKEN

SERVES
8

PREP TIME
8
HOURS

COOK TIME
10
MINUTES

- **1 pound** chicken tender

- **2** green onions, chopped

- **1/2 cup** fat-free low sodium chicken broth

- **1/4 cup** sherry cooking wine

- **3 tablespoons** low sodium soy sauce

- **1 tablespoon** grated ginger

- **2 cloves** garlic, minced

1. In a large resealable bag, add all ingredients. Seal and shake the bag to mix well. Marinate overnight.

2. Preheat the broiler. Thread the meat onto 16 skewers.

3. Broil 3-4 minutes on each side.

CALORIES	CARBS	SUGAR	FAT	PROTEIN	SODIUM
64	1.1	0.2	0.3	11.6	343
KCAL	GRAMS	GRAMS	GRAMS	GRAMS	MILLIGRAMS

TUNA POKE

 SERVES
4

 PREP TIME
5
MINUTES

 COOK TIME
5
MINUTES

1. In a medium bowl, combine all ingredients and serve.

- **1/2 pound** sushi grade tuna, cubed

- **1/4 cup** finely chopped green onion

- **2 tablespoons** low sodium soy sauce

- **1 teaspoon** lime juice

- **1 teaspoon** roasted sesame seed

CALORIES	CARBS	SUGAR	FAT	PROTEIN	SODIUM
91	1.0	0.0	2.4	14.7	310
KCAL	GRAMS	GRAMS	GRAMS	GRAMS	MILLIGRAMS

BROILED CURRY SALMON

SERVES
4

PREP TIME
10
MINUTES

COOK TIME
10
MINUTES

- **2** salmon fillets (6-ounce each)
- **1 teaspoon** curry powder
- **1 teaspoon** garlic powder
- **1/2 teaspoon** cumin
- **1/4 teaspoon** salt

1. Preheat the broiler.

2. Mix the spice in a small bowl. Rub the spice evenly on the salmon.

3. Broil for 8-12 minutes.

CALORIES	CARBS	SUGAR	FAT	PROTEIN	SODIUM
80	0.9	0.0	0.9	18.2	256
KCAL	GRAMS	GRAMS	GRAMS	GRAMS	MILLIGRAMS

PORTOBELLO TUNA MELT

SERVES
4

PREP TIME
5
MINUTES

COOK TIME
20
MINUTES

1. Preheat the broiler

2. In a medium bowl, combine tuna, mayonnaise, sour cream, onion and season with salt and pepper

3. Divide the tuna mixture on the mushroom.

4. Place a slice of tomato on each mushroom. Then Top with mozzarella cheese.

5. Place the mushroom on a rack and broil for 10-15 minutes until the cheese turns golden brown.

- 4 Portobello Mushroom, Gills and stems removed

- **1** 5-ounce **can** tuna in water, drained

- **4 slices** tomatoes

- **1/4 cup** chopped onion

- **1/4 cup** low fat mayonnaise

- **1/4 cup** fat-free sour cream

- **1/4 cup** fat-free parmesan cheese

- **3/4 cup** fat-free mozzarella cheese

- salt and pepper to taste

CALORIES	CARBS	SUGAR	FAT	PROTEIN	SODIUM
137	14.8	3.7	1.8	17.5	620
KCAL	GRAMS	GRAMS	GRAMS	GRAMS	MILLIGRAMS

BUFFALO RANCH SALMON

 SERVES **4**

 PREP TIME **10** MINUTES

 COOK TIME **15** MINUTES

- **2** salmon fillets (6-ounce each)
- **2 tablespoon** whole wheat breadcrumbs
- **2 tablespoons** buffalo sauce
- **1 tablespoons** fat-free ranch seasoning
- **1/4 teaspoon** salt
- **1/4 teaspoon** pepper

1. Preheat the oven to 425°F.

2. In a small bowl, combine buffalo sauce, ranch seasoning, salt and pepper.

3. Spread the sauce on each salmon fillets. Sprinkle the breadcrumbs on top of each fillet.

4. Bake for 15 minutes.

CALORIES	CARBS	SUGAR	FAT	PROTEIN	SODIUM
95	2.6	0.4	1.6	18.4	469
KCAL	GRAMS	GRAMS	GRAMS	GRAMS	MILLIGRAMS

LEMON GLAZED SALMON

 SERVES 4

 PREP TIME 5 MINUTES

 COOK TIME 20 MINUTES

1. Brown the salmon fillet. Set aside.

2. Sauté garlic until fragrant.

3. Add lemon zest, lemon juice and broth. Simmer on low until reduces by half. Season with salt and pepper.

4. Return the Salmon. Simmer until the salmon is cooked through. Sprinkle parsley and serve.

- 2 salmon fillets (6-ounce each)
- 1 lemon, thinly sliced
- **2 tablespoons** lemon juice
- **1 tablespoon** lemon zest
- **3 cloves** garlic, minced
- **1 cup** fat-free low sodium chicken broth
- **2 tablespoons** chopped fresh parsley
- salt and pepper to taste
- Non-stick Cooking Spray

CALORIES	CARBS	SUGAR	FAT	PROTEIN	SODIUM
83	1.8	0.2	0.8	18.7	132
KCAL	GRAMS	GRAMS	GRAMS	GRAMS	MILLIGRAMS

SMOKED SALMON SCRAMBLE

 SERVES
8

 PREP TIME
10
MINUTES

 COOK TIME
15
MINUTES

- **4 ounces** smoked salmon

- **2** large eggs and **4** egg whites

- **2 cups** baby spinach

- **2 cloves** garlic, minced

- **2 tablespoons** low fat cheddar cheese

- salt and pepper to taste

- Nonstick Cooking Spray

1. Sauté garlic and spinach until fragrant.

2. In a medium bowl, whisk the eggs and cheese. Season with salt and pepper.

3. Add the egg mixture. Scramble for 30 seconds.

4. Add salmon. Scramble for until eggs are cooked through.

CALORIES	CARBS	SUGAR	FAT	PROTEIN	SODIUM
97	1.4	0.4	3.9	13.1	320
KCAL	GRAMS	GRAMS	GRAMS	GRAMS	MILLIGRAMS

TILAPIA TOMATO ALFREDO

 SERVES
8

 PREP TIME
5
MINUTES

 COOK TIME
20
MINUTES

1. Season the fish with salt and pepper. Set aside.

2. Sauté garlic and onion until fragrant.

3. Add soup, milk and tomatoes. Cook until bubbly. Add Fish and bring it to a boil. Then reduce to low and simmer for 10-15 minutes.

- **1 pound** tilapia fillet, cut into 2-inch pieces

- **1** 10.5-ounce **can** fat-free condensed cream of mushroom soup

- **1** 10-ounce **can** diced tomatoes, drained

- **1/2 cup** chopped onion

- **3 cloves** garlic, minced

- **1/2 cup** skim milk

- **2 tablespoons** chopped fresh parsley

- salt and pepper to taste

- Nonstick Cooking Spray

CALORIES	CARBS	SUGAR	FAT	PROTEIN	SODIUM
84	**5.8**	**1.8**	**2.1**	**11.3**	**324**
KCAL	GRAMS	GRAMS	GRAMS	GRAMS	MILLIGRAMS

SPICY HALIBUT PARMESAN

 SERVES
8

 PREP TIME
15
MINUTES

 COOK TIME
10
MINUTES

- **1 pound** skinless halibut fillets

- **1** green onion, chopped

- **1/2 cup** fat-free parmesan cheese

- **1 1/2 tablespoons** fat-free mayonnaise

- **1 tablespoons** lemon juice

- **1 teaspoon** hot sauce

- **1/4 teaspoon** salt

- Nonstick Cooking Spray

1. Preheat the oven to 425°F.

2. In a medium bowl, combine all ingredients except fish.

3. Season the fish with salt and pepper. Place the fish on a baking dish. Bake for 10 minutes.

4. Spread the cheese mixture on top and bake for another 5 minutes or until cheese are bubbly and golden brown.

CALORIES	CARBS	SUGAR	FAT	PROTEIN	SODIUM
68	3.8	0.3	0.5	12.5	270
KCAL	GRAMS	GRAMS	GRAMS	GRAMS	MILLIGRAMS

ASIAN SALMON MEATBALLS

SERVES 6	PREP TIME 5 MINUTES	COOK TIME 25 MINUTES

1. Preheat the oven to 350°F.

2. In a large bowl, combine all ingredients. Divide the mixture into 12 meatballs. Apply nonstick cooking spray.

3. Bake for 15-18 minutes.

- **12 ounces** canned pink salmon, drained

- **1/2 cup** whole wheat breadcrumbs

- **2** green onions, finely chopped

- **2 cloves** garlic, minced

- **1/2 tablespoon** grated ginger

- **1** egg

- **1/4 teaspoon** salt

- **1/4 teaspoon** ground black pepper

CALORIES	CARBS	SUGAR	FAT	PROTEIN	SODIUM
99 KCAL	5.6 GRAMS	0.5 GRAMS	2.5 GRAMS	14.2 GRAMS	296 MILLIGRAMS

SPICY PEANUT SALMON BURGER

SERVES
6

PREP TIME
5
MINUTES

COOK TIME
25
MINUTES

- **12 ounces** canned pink salmon, drained

- **1/2 cup** whole wheat breadcrumbs

- **2** green onions, finely chopped

- **1 1/2 tablespoons** low sodium soy sauce

- **2 tablespoons** powdered peanut butter

- **1 tablespoon** hot sauce

- **1/4 cup** fat-free Greek yogurt

1. Preheat the oven to 350°F.

2. In a large bowl, combine all ingredients. Divide the mixture into 12 patties. Apply nonstick cooking spray.

3. Bake for 15-18 minutes.

CALORIES	CARBS	SUGAR	FAT	PROTEIN	SODIUM
120	7.0	0.9	3.4	16.1	477
KCAL	GRAMS	GRAMS	GRAMS	GRAMS	MILLIGRAMS

ASIAN GINGER CATFISH

SERVES
8

PREP TIME
15
MINUTES

COOK TIME
20
MINUTES

1. Sauté ginger until golden brown. Sear the fish. 3 minutes on each side. Set aside.

2. Sauté garlic, green onion, onion and bell peppers until fragrant. Add fish sauce, soy sauce and oyster sauce. Return the fish and bury the fish in the sauce and cook for 3-5 more minutes.

- **1 pound** catfish fillet, cut into 2-inch pieces
- **4 ounces** fresh ginger, peeled and cut into thin strips
- **1/2 cup** chopped onion
- **1/2 cup** sliced red bell peppers
- **2** green onions, chopped
- **2 tablespoons** fish sauce
- **1 tablespoons** oyster sauce
- **1 tablespoon** low-sodium soy sauce
- Nonstick Cooking Spray

CALORIES	CARBS	SUGAR	FAT	PROTEIN	SODIUM
123	**3.5**	**1.2**	**1.0**	**12.3**	**518**
KCAL	GRAMS	GRAMS	GRAMS	GRAMS	MILLIGRAMS

CHEESY TUNA CASSEROLE

 SERVES
8

 PREP TIME
10
MINUTES

 COOK TIME
30
MINUTES

- **3** 5-ounce **cans** tuna in water, drained

- **1** medium head cauliflower, cut into florets

- **1 cup** diced onion

- **1 cup** low-fat alfredo sauce

- **1 cup** skim milk

- **1/2 cup** fat-free parmesan cheese

- **1 cup** fat-free mozzarella cheese

- Nonstick Cooking Spray

1. Preheat the broiler

2. In a large pot, add enough water to cover the cauliflower. Cook until cauliflower is soft. Drain and mash the cauliflower. Season with salt and pepper.

3. Sauté onion until fragrant. Add milk and alfredo sauce. Stir in the parmesan cheese, tuna and cauliflower mash. Adjust seasoning if needed.

4. Top with mozzarella cheese and broil until the cheese is golden brown and bubbly.

CALORIES	CARBS	SUGAR	FAT	PROTEIN	SODIUM
148	12.0	4.2	3.5	18.0	670
KCAL	GRAMS	GRAMS	GRAMS	GRAMS	MILLIGRAMS

MEDITERRANEAN WHITE FISH

SERVES
8

PREP TIME
15
MINUTES

COOK TIME
30
MINUTES

1. Preheat the oven to 425°F.

2. Season the fish with salt and pepper. Place the fish on a baking dish. Set aside.

3. Sauté garlic and onion until fragrant. Then add tomatoes and cook until tender. Add capers, olives, wine, oregano and basil. Reduce to low heat. Stir in cheese. Cook on low until the sauce reduces by half.

4. Spread the sauce on the fish. Bake for 10-15 minutes.

- **1 pound** white fish fillet
- **5** plum tomatoes, diced
- **1/2 cup** chopped onion
- **2 cloves** garlic, minced
- **4 tablespoons** capers
- **6** black olives, pitted and chopped
- **1/4 cup** dry white wine
- **3 tablespoons** fat-free parmesan cheese
- **1/2 teaspoon** dried basil
- pinch of dried oregano

CALORIES	CARBS	SUGAR	FAT	PROTEIN	SODIUM
98	3.8	1.8	1.3	14.8	340
KCAL	GRAMS	GRAMS	GRAMS	GRAMS	MILLIGRAMS

GARLIC HERB TUNA STEAK

 SERVES
4

 PREP TIME
40
MINUTES

 COOK TIME
10
MINUTES

- **2** tuna steak (6-ounce each)
- **2 cloves** garlic, minced
- **2 tablespoons** lemon juice
- **2 teaspoons** minced fresh thyme
- **1/4 teaspoon** salt
- **1/4 teaspoon** pepper

1. In a large resealable plastic bag, combine all ingredients. Put in the refrigerator and marinade for 30 minutes.

2. Preheat the broiler.

3. Discard the marinade, broil the tuna steak 3-4 minutes on each side.

CALORIES	CARBS	SUGAR	FAT	PROTEIN	SODIUM
95	1.3	0.2	0.8	19.7	173
KCAL	GRAMS	GRAMS	GRAMS	GRAMS	MILLIGRAMS

SPICY HUMMUS TUNA CAKE

 SERVES
12

 PREP TIME
20
MINUTES

 COOK TIME
40
MINUTES

1. Preheat the oven to 350°F.

2. In a large bowl, combine all ingredients.

3. Spray a muffin tin. Divide the mixture into 12 cups.

4. Bake for 40 minutes.

- **3** 5-ounce **cans** tuna in water, drained
- **1 cup** roasted red pepper hummus
- **2 cloves** garlic, minced
- **1** green onion, chopped
- **1** jalapeno pepper, seeded and chopped
- **2** large eggs
- **1/4 teaspoon** salt

CALORIES	CARBS	SUGAR	FAT	PROTEIN	SODIUM
85	4.3	0.1	3.8	8.7	312
KCAL	GRAMS	GRAMS	GRAMS	GRAMS	MILLIGRAMS

BALSAMIC PORK TENDERLOIN

 SERVES
6

 PREP TIME
15
MINUTES

 COOK TIME
10
MINUTES

- **1 pound** pork tenderloin, cut into 1.5-inch piece

- **1/4 cup** fat-free low sodium chicken broth

- **2 tablespoons** balsamic vinegar

- **2 tablespoons** whole wheat flour

- **1 teaspoon** capers

- **1 teaspoon** lemon zest

- **1/2 teaspoon** salt

- **1/4 teaspoon** pepper

1. In a small bowl, mix together flour, salt and pepper. Coat the pork in the mixture. Shake off excess flour.

2. Brown the pork. Add vinegar and broth. Bring to a boil and reduce to low. Simmer for 4-5 minutes until pork is cooked through.

3. Remove the pork. Add lemon zest and capers. Simmer until the desired consistency. Pour the sauce over the pork and serve.

CALORIES	CARBS	SUGAR	FAT	PROTEIN	SODIUM
77	2.7	0.8	1.4	15.0	550
KCAL	GRAMS	GRAMS	GRAMS	GRAMS	MILLIGRAMS

PORK AND BROCCOLI STIR FRY

SERVES
8

PREP TIME
5
MINUTES

COOK TIME
20
MINUTES

1. In a large bowl, mix the pork with soy sauce, garlic, ground ginger and crushed red pepper. Set aside to marinate.

2. Blanch the broccoli in a pot of boiling water until slightly softened. Drain and set aside.

3. Sauté onion until fragrant. Set aside.

4. Add the pork without the marinate. Cook until cook through.

5. Dissolve the flour in the broth. Add broth and sauce. Cook until sauce thickens.

6. Add the broccoli and onion. Stir fry for 2-3 minutes until cooked through.

- **1 pound** pork tenderloin, thinly sliced

- **12 ounces** broccoli floret

- **1 cup** sliced onion

- **2 cloves** garlic, minced

- **1 cup** fat free low sodium chicken broth

- **2 tablespoons** low sodium soy sauce

- **1 tablespoon** whole wheat flour

- **1/4 teaspoon** ground ginger

- **1/8 teaspoon** crushed red pepper

- Nonstick Cooking Spray

CALORIES	CARBS	SUGAR	FAT	PROTEIN	SODIUM
78	6.0	1.3	1.2	13.0	364
KCAL	GRAMS	GRAMS	GRAMS	GRAMS	MILLIGRAMS

PORK CHOPS IN MUSHROOM SAUCE

 SERVES
8

 PREP TIME
10
MINUTES

 COOK TIME
40
MINUTES

- **4** pork chops (4-ounce each)
- **1** 10.5-ounce **can** fat-free condensed cream of mushroom soup
- **2 cups** sliced mushrooms
- **1 cup** chopped onion
- **2 cloves** garlic, minced
- **2 tablespoons** dry white wine
- pinch of thyme
- salt and pepper to taste
- Nonstick Cooking Spray

1. Season the pork chops with salt and pepper.

2. Sauté garlic and onion until fragrant. Set aside.

3. Brown the pork chops. Add all ingredients and mix well. Cover and simmer on low for 20-25 minutes

CALORIES	CARBS	SUGAR	FAT	PROTEIN	SODIUM
107	6.0	0.9	3.1	13.1	521
KCAL	GRAMS	GRAMS	GRAMS	GRAMS	MILLIGRAMS

PORK CHOPS IN CREAMY ONION SAUCE

 SERVES
8

 PREP TIME
10
MINUTES

 COOK TIME
40
MINUTES

1. Season the pork chops with salt and pepper.

2. Sauté garlic and onion until fragrant. Set aside.

3. Brown the pork chops. Add broth. Cover and simmer on low for 20-25 minutes.

4. Remove the pork chops. Simmer the sauce until reduces by half. Stir in sour cream and paprika. Pour the sauce over the pork chops and serve.

- 4 pork chops (4-ounce each)

- **1 1/2 cups** chopped onion

- **1/2 cup** fat-free low sodium chicken broth

- **1 clove** garlic, minced

- **3/4 cup** fat-free sour cream

- **2 teaspoons** paprika

- salt and pepper to taste

- Nonstick Cooking Spray

CALORIES	CARBS	SUGAR	FAT	PROTEIN	SODIUM
95	5.5	2.8	2.4	13.6	153
KCAL	GRAMS	GRAMS	GRAMS	GRAMS	MILLIGRAMS

PORK STROGANOFF

 SERVES
8

 PREP TIME
10
MINUTES

 COOK TIME
40
MINUTES

- **1 pound** pork tenderloin, cut into thin strips
- **2 cups** sliced mushrooms
- **1 cup** chopped onion
- **2 cloves** garlic, minced
- **1/2 cup** fat-free low-sodium chicken broth
- **1 cup** fat-free half and half
- **2 tablespoons** fat free sour cream
- **1 tablespoon** mustard
- **1 teaspoon** paprika
- **1 teaspoon** tomato paste
- **1 teaspoon** chili powder
- **1 teaspoon** lemon juice
- salt and pepper to taste

1. Season the pork chops with salt and pepper.

2. Sauté garlic, onion and mushrooms until fragrant. Set aside.

3. Brown the pork chops. Add broth. Cover and simmer on low for 20-25 minutes.

4. Remove the pork chops.

5. Stir in cream, mustard, tomato paste, lemon juice and other seasoning. Pour the sauce over the pork

CALORIES	CARBS	SUGAR	FAT	PROTEIN	SODIUM
93	7.3	2.7	1.5	13.6	448
KCAL	GRAMS	GRAMS	GRAMS	GRAMS	MILLIGRAMS

VINEGAR MUSTARD GLAZED HAM LOAF

 SERVES **16**

 PREP TIME **10** MINUTES

 COOK TIME **90** MINUTES

1. Preheat the oven to 350°F.

2. In a large bowl, combine ham, pork, eggs, evaporated milk, salt and pepper. Spray a 9x13 baking dish. Place the mixture in the dish. Bake for 90 minutes.

3. In a small bowl, mix together vinegar, mustard and truvia. Pour the mixture on top of the loaf in the last 15 minutes.

- **2 pounds** extra lean ham
- **1 pound** extra lean ground pork
- **2 eggs**
- **1 cup** whole wheat breadcrumbs
- **1 cup** low-fat evaporated milk
- **1/3 cup** Truvia brown sugar
- **1/4 cup** apple cider vinegar
- **1 tablespoon** mustard powder
- **1/4 teaspoon** salt
- **1/4 teaspoon** ground black pepper

CALORIES	CARBS	SUGAR	FAT	PROTEIN	SODIUM
146	9.6	4.3	4.7	17.3	755
KCAL	GRAMS	GRAMS	GRAMS	GRAMS	MILLIGRAMS

GARLIC LEMON SCALLOPS

 SERVES
8

 PREP TIME
5
MINUTES

 COOK TIME
10
MINUTES

- **1 pound** sea scallops, patted dry

- **6 cloves** garlic, minced

- **2 scallions**, finely chopped

- **1 lemon**, juice only

- **1 tablespoon** whole wheat flour

- **1/4 teaspoon** salt

- pinch of ground sage

- Nonstick cooking spray

1. In a bowl, mix scallops with flour and salt.

2. Spray a large skillet, Sear the scallops until golden brown. Set aside.

3. sauté garlic and scallion until fragrant. Add lemon juice and return scallops. Stir well and cook for 30 seconds. Sprinkle with parsley and serve.

CALORIES	CARBS	SUGAR	FAT	PROTEIN	SODIUM
72	5.2	0.2	0.5	11.7	450
KCAL	GRAMS	GRAMS	GRAMS	GRAMS	MILLIGRAMS

SCALLOPS IN JALAPENO WHISKY CREAM SAUCE

SERVES
8

PREP TIME
5
MINUTES

COOK TIME
10
MINUTES

1. In a bowl, mix scallops with flour and 1/4 teaspoon salt. Spray a large skillet, Sear the scallops until golden brown. Set aside.

2. sauté garlic and pepper until fragrant. Add whisky and cook for 1 minute. Stir in cream and bring to a simmer. Season with salt and pepper.

3. Pour sauce over scallops. Sprinkle with chopped cilantro and serve.

- **1 pound** sea scallops, patted dry

- **2 cloves** garlic, minced

- **2** jalapeno pepper, seeded and finely chopped

- **1 cup** fat-free half and half

- **1/2 cup** chopped fresh cilantro

- **1/8 cup** bourbon whiskey

- **1 tablespoon** whole wheat flour

- **3/4 teaspoon** salt

- **1/2 teaspoon** ground black pepper

CALORIES	CARBS	SUGAR	FAT	PROTEIN	SODIUM
96	7.1	1.7	0.9	12.4	623
KCAL	GRAMS	GRAMS	GRAMS	GRAMS	MILLIGRAMS

LOWCOUNTRY SHRIMPS

 SERVES
8

 PREP TIME
5
MINUTES

 COOK TIME
15
MINUTES

- **1 pound** fresh shrimps, peeled and deveined

- **1** 6.5-ounce **link** lean turkey sausage, sliced

- **1 cup** sliced bell pepper

- **2 cloves** garlic, minced

- **1 teaspoon** old bay seasoning

- **1/4 teaspoon** ground black pepper

- **1/4 cup** water

- Nonstick Cooking Spray

1. In a large bowl, season shrimp with old bay seasoning and black pepper. Set aside.

2. Spray a large skillet, sauté garlic until fragrant. Add sausage and cook until crispy. Add shrimp and water. Cook while stirring until cook through.

CALORIES	CARBS	SUGAR	FAT	PROTEIN	SODIUM
75	1.2	0.4	1.6	13.5	448
KCAL	GRAMS	GRAMS	GRAMS	GRAMS	MILLIGRAMS

CHEESY ONION SCALLOPS

SERVES
8

PREP TIME
5
MINUTES

COOK TIME
15
MINUTES

1. Preheat the broiler.

2. In a bowl, mix scallops with flour and 1/4 teaspoon salt. Spray an oven-proof skillet. Sear the scallops until golden brown. Set aside.

3. sauté garlic, onion and shallots until fragrant. Add wine and water. Simmer until the sauce reduces by half. Season with salt and pepper.

4. Stir in the scallops. Top with cheese and broil for 3-5 minutes until cheese turns golden brown.

- **1 pound** sea scallops, patted dry
- **2 cloves** garlic, minced
- **2** shallots, chopped
- **1/4 cup** chopped onion
- **3/4 cup** white wine
- **1/4 cup** water
- **1/4 cup** fat-free parmesan cheese
- **1** bay leave
- **2 tablespoons** chopped fresh thyme
- **1 tablespoon** whole wheat flour
- salt and pepper to taste

CALORIES	CARBS	SUGAR	FAT	PROTEIN	SODIUM
94	**6.0**	**0.3**	**0.5**	**12.1**	**460**
KCAL	GRAMS	GRAMS	GRAMS	GRAMS	MILLIGRAMS

SHRIMP À LA GRECQUE

 SERVES
8

 PREP TIME
5
MINUTES

 COOK TIME
20
MINUTES

- **1 pound** fresh shrimps, peeled and deveined

- **1 1/2 cups** canned crushed tomatoes, drained

- **3 ounces** fat-free feta cheese, cubed

- **2 cloves** garlic, minced

- **1/2 cup** dry white wine

- **2 tablespoons** chopped fresh parsley

- **1/2 teaspoon** dried oregano, crushed

- **1/4 teaspoon** salt

- **1/4 teaspoon** ground black pepper

1. Spray a large skillet, sauté garlic until fragrant. Add tomatoes, wine, oregano, salt and pepper. Cook until sauce thickens.

2. Add shrimp, cook while stirring until cook through. Remove from heat. Add cheese and parsley before serving.

CALORIES	CARBS	SUGAR	FAT	PROTEIN	SODIUM
97	4.3	1.7	0.9	14.1	507
KCAL	GRAMS	GRAMS	GRAMS	GRAMS	MILLIGRAMS

CRAB IMPERIAL

SERVES
8

PREP TIME
10
MINUTES

COOK TIME
20
MINUTES

1. Preheat the oven to 400°F.

2. In a large bowl, combine all

3. ingredients except paprika and cilantro.

4. Transfer the mixture to a baking dish. Sprinkle Paprika and bake for 20 minutes. Garnish with fresh cilantro and serve.

- **1 pound** crab meat
- **1/2 cup** chopped bell peppers
- **1/2 cup** chopped celery
- **2** egg whites, beaten
- **1/2** lemon, juice only
- **1 cup** fat-free plain yogurt
- **2 tablespoons** chopped fresh cilantro
- **1 teaspoon** dry mustard
- **1/4 teaspoon** salt
- **1/4 teaspoon** Worcestershire sauce
- **1/8 teaspoon** chili powder
- **1/8 teaspoon** paprika

CALORIES	CARBS	SUGAR	FAT	PROTEIN	SODIUM
76	10.8	4.9	0.6	7.4	423
KCAL	GRAMS	GRAMS	GRAMS	GRAMS	MILLIGRAMS

STEAMED CLAMS IN GARLIC WINE SAUCE

 SERVES 5

 PREP TIME 10 MINUTES

 COOK TIME 25 MINUTES

- **50** small clams, scrubbed
- **1 cup** white wine
- **8 cloves** garlic, minced
- **1/2 cup** chopped fresh parsley
- **1 tablespoon** butter
- salt and pepper to taste
- Nonstick Cooking Spray

1. Spray a large skillet, sauté garlic until fragrant. Add wine. Simmer until sauce reduces by half, about 15 minutes.

2. Add clams, cover and steam until clams begin to open, about 5 minutes.

3. Stir in butter and cover. Steam until most clams open, about 5 minutes. Season with salt and pepper. Sprinkle with parsley and serve.

CALORIES	CARBS	SUGAR	FAT	PROTEIN	SODIUM
168	5.7	0.1	3.6	18.9	111
KCAL	GRAMS	GRAMS	GRAMS	GRAMS	MILLIGRAMS

MUSSELS IN MARINARA SAUCE

SERVES
6

PREP TIME
10
MINUTES

COOK TIME
30
MINUTES

1. Spray a large skillet, sauté garlic until fragrant. Add wine. Simmer until sauce reduces by half, about 15 minutes.

2. Add tomatoes and green onion and cook for 4-5 minutes until softens.

3. Add mussels. Cover and cook until mussels start to open, about 5 minutes. Stir in butter. cover and cook until most mussels open.

4. Sprinkle with parsley and serve.

- **50** mussels, scrubbed and debearded

- **6 cloves** garlic, minced

- **3** plum tomatoes, chopped

- **3** green onion, chopped

- **1/2 cup** chopped fresh parsley

- **1 cup** white wine

- **1 tablespoon** butter

- salt and pepper to taste

- Nonstick Cooking Spray

CALORIES	CARBS	SUGAR	FAT	PROTEIN	SODIUM
174	**8.1**	**1.3**	**4.9**	**16.9**	**410**
KCAL	GRAMS	GRAMS	GRAMS	GRAMS	MILLIGRAMS

CREAMY CAJUN SHRIMPS

 SERVES
12

 PREP TIME
10
MINUTES

 COOK TIME
30
MINUTES

- **1 1/2 pounds** fresh shrimps, peeled and deveined

- **1/2 cup** sliced mushrooms

- **2** green onions, chopped

- **1/4 cup** low-fat alfredo sauce

- **1/4 cup** chopped fresh parsley

- **1/4 cup** skim milk

- **1/4 cup** fat-free grated parmesan cheese

- **1 tablespoon** Cajun seasoning

- salt and pepper to taste

- Nonstick Cooking Spray

1. Preheat the oven to 350°F.

2. Season the shrimp with Cajun seasoning, salt and pepper.

3. Spray a large skillet, sauté mushrooms and green onion until fragrant. Add shrimp and sauté until cooked through. Transfer to a baking Dish.

4. Add alfredo sauce and skim milk to the pan and stir to combine.

   Pour the sauce over the shrimps. Sprinkle with parmesan cheese and bake for 20 minutes.

CALORIES	CARBS	SUGAR	FAT	PROTEIN	SODIUM
69	1.2	0.4	1.3	12.7	485
KCAL	GRAMS	GRAMS	GRAMS	GRAMS	MILLIGRAMS

MARYLAND CRAB CAKE

 SERVES
8

 PREP TIME
60
MINUTES

 COOK TIME
15
MINUTES

1. In a large bowl, combine crabmeat, egg, half of the breadcrumbs, mayonnaise, mustard, Worcestershire sauce and all seasoning. Refrigerate for 1 hour.

2. Spread the remaining breadcrumbs on a large plate.

3. Divide the crab mixture into 8 portions and shape into patties. Coat with bread crumbs on each side.

4. Spray a pan, cook the crab cakes until golden brown on each side.

- **1 pound** crab meat

- **1/2 cup** whole wheat breadcrumbs, divided

- **2 tablespoons** fat-free mayonnaise

- **1 egg**, beaten

- **1/2 teaspoon** Dijon Mustard

- **1/2 teaspoon** Old Bay seasoning

- **1/4 teaspoon** Worcestershire sauce

- **1/4 teaspoon** salt

- **1/8 teaspoon** ground black pepper

- Nonstick cooking spray

CALORIES	CARBS	SUGAR	FAT	PROTEIN	SODIUM
69	4.1	0.6	0.7	11.5	346
KCAL	GRAMS	GRAMS	GRAMS	GRAMS	MILLIGRAMS

GRILLED TOMATO BASIL SHRIMPS

 SERVES
8

 PREP TIME
2
HOURS

 COOK TIME
15
MINUTES

- **1 pound** fresh shrimps, peeled and deveined

- **4 cloves** garlic, minced

- **3 tablespoons** tomato sauce

- **2 tablespoons** chopped fresh basil

- **1 tablespoons** red wine vinegar

- **1 tablespoon** olive oil

- **1/4 teaspoon** salt

- **1/8 teaspoon** cayenne pepper

- Nonstick Cooking Spray

1. In a large resealable bag, add all ingredients and mix well. Seal the bag and refrigerate for 2 hours to marinate.

2. Prepare the grill. Thread the shrimp onto skewers. Spray the Grill. Cook shrimp for 2-3 minutes on each side or until opaque

CALORIES	CARBS	SUGAR	FAT	PROTEIN	SODIUM
77	0.9	0.5	2.6	12.2	361
KCAL	GRAMS	GRAMS	GRAMS	GRAMS	MILLIGRAMS

GRILLED LEMON GINGER SHRIMPS

SERVES
8

PREP TIME
10
MINUTES

COOK TIME
50
MINUTES

1. In a large resealable bag, add all ingredients and mix well. Seal the bag and refrigerate for 2 hours to marinate.

2. Prepare the grill. Thread the shrimp onto skewers. Spray the Grill. Cook shrimp for 2-3 minutes on each side or until opaque

- **1 pound** fresh shrimps, peeled and deveined

- **4 cloves** garlic, minced

- **1/4 cup** lemon juice

- **1/4 cup** chopped fresh cilantro

- **3 tablespoons** grated ginger

- **1 teaspoon** paprika

- **1/4 teaspoon** salt

- **1/4 teaspoon** ground black pepper

CALORIES	CARBS	SUGAR	FAT	PROTEIN	SODIUM
66	1.9	0.3	1.0	12.4	345
KCAL	GRAMS	GRAMS	GRAMS	GRAMS	MILLIGRAMS

TACO SALAD

 SERVES
8

 PREP TIME
15
MINUTES

 COOK TIME
10
MINUTES

- **1 pound** 97/3 lean ground beef

- **1 head** romaine lettuce, chopped

- **2** medium tomatoes, chopped

- **8** green onions, green and white separated and chopped

- **1 1/2 cups** fat-free shredded cheddar cheese

- **1/2 cup** fat-free Greek Yogurt

- **1/2 cup** salsa

- **1 tablespoon** chili powder

- salt and pepper to taste

1. Brown the beef with white part of onions. Season with chili powder, salt and pepper.

2. In a large bowl, toss all ingredients except yogurt and salsa together. Spoon yogurt and salsa on the side and serve.

CALORIES	CARBS	SUGAR	FAT	PROTEIN	SODIUM
134	7.6	2.7	2.4	21.8	376
KCAL	GRAMS	GRAMS	GRAMS	GRAMS	MILLIGRAMS

ASIAN LETTUCE WRAP

 SERVES
8

 PREP TIME
15
MINUTES

 COOK TIME
20
MINUTES

1. Spray a large skillet, sauté garlic, onion, green onion and water chestnut until fragrant. Drain the liquid and set aside.

2. Brown the beef. Then add all ingredients except lettuce. Stir well. Cook for another 2-3 minutes.

3. Divide the beef onto the lettuce leaves. Roll up and serve.

- **1 pound** 97/3 lean ground beef
- **1** 8-ounce **can** water chestnut, finely chopped
- **8** large romaine lettuce leaves
- **2 cloves** garlic, minced
- **1/2 cup** chopped onion
- **1/4 cup** chopped green onion
- **1/4 cup** hoisin sauce
- **2 tablespoons** low sodium soy sauce
- **2 tablespoon** rice wine vinegar
- **1 tablespoon** chili paste
- **1 tablespoon** grated ginger
- **1 tablespoon** sesame oil
- Nonstick cooking spray

CALORIES	CARBS	SUGAR	FAT	PROTEIN	SODIUM
121	9.0	3.5	4.1	13.0	351
KCAL	GRAMS	GRAMS	GRAMS	GRAMS	MILLIGRAMS

SHRIMP SALAD STUFFED TOMATOES

 SERVES
8

 PREP TIME
35
MINUTES

 COOK TIME
/
MINUTES

- **1 pound** shrimp, peeled, deveined, cooked and chopped

- **4** large ripe tomatoes, cored

- **1 stalk** celery, chopped

- **1** shallot, minced

- **1/4 cup** chopped fresh basil

- **2 tablespoons** low-fat mayonnaise

- **1 tablespoon** white wine vinegar

- salt and pepper to taste

- pinch of paprika

1. In a medium bowl, combine shrimp, celery, shallots, basil, mayonnaise and vinegar. Season with salt and pepper.

2. Spoon the mixture into the tomatoes. Garnish with pinch of paprika and serve.

CALORIES	CARBS	SUGAR	FAT	PROTEIN	SODIUM
80	4.5	2.8	1.3	12.9	309
KCAL	GRAMS	GRAMS	GRAMS	GRAMS	MILLIGRAMS

SLOPPY JOE LETTUCE WRAP

SERVES
8

PREP TIME
10
MINUTES

COOK TIME
40
MINUTES

1. Spray a large skillet, sauté garlic, onion and bell pepper until fragrant. Drain the liquid and set aside.

2. Brown the beef. Then add all ingredients except lettuce. Stir well. Reduce to low heat and simmer for 25 minutes.

3. Divide the beef onto the lettuce leaves. Roll up and serve.

- **1 pound** 97/3 lean ground beef
- **8** large romaine lettuce leaves
- **3/4 cup** tomato sauce
- **1/4 cup** chopped onion
- **1/4 cup** chopped green bell peppers
- **2 cloves** garlic, minced.
- **1 teaspoon** yellow mustard
- **1 teaspoon** stevia
- salt and pepper to taste
- Nonstick Cooking Spray

CALORIES	CARBS	SUGAR	FAT	PROTEIN	SODIUM
82	3.6	1.6	2.2	12.8	155
KCAL	GRAMS	GRAMS	GRAMS	GRAMS	MILLIGRAMS

GARDEN SALAD WITH LEMON CHICKEN AND FETA

 SERVES
6

 PREP TIME
40
MINUTES

 COOK TIME
20
MINUTES

For Chicken:

- 2 boneless skinless chicken breasts
- 1/4 cup lemon juice
- 2 cloves garlic, minced
- 2 tablespoons chopped fresh dill
- 1/2 teaspoon salt
- 1/4 teaspoon ground black pepper
- Nonstick cooking spray

For salad:

- 1/2 medium seedless cucumber, chopped
- 2 medium tomatoes, chopped
- 3 ounces fat-free feta cheese, cubed
- 2 tablespoons lemon juice
- 1 tablespoon olive oil
- 1/2 teaspoon Dijon mustard
- 1/2 teaspoon stevia
- salt and pepper to taste

1. In a medium resealable bag, add all ingredients for the chicken. Seal and press to coat the marinade evenly. Refrigerate for 30 minutes. Discard the marinade and dry the chicken.

2. Sear the chicken until golden brown on one side. Flip, reduce to low heat, cover and cook for 10-15 minutes until cooked through. Set aside to cool. Then slice into bite size.

3. Combine lemon juice, olive oil, mustard and stevia. In a large bowl, toss all ingredients together and serve.

CALORIES	CARBS	SUGAR	FAT	PROTEIN	SODIUM
111	8.5	3.1	2.9	12.9	475
KCAL	GRAMS	GRAMS	GRAMS	GRAMS	MILLIGRAMS

BUFFALO CHICKEN LETTUCE WRAP

 SERVES
8

 PREP TIME
10
MINUTES

 COOK TIME
60
MINUTES

1. Brown the chicken tender on both sides.

2. Add broth and beer. Cover and simmer for 1 hour.

3. Shredd the chicken. Add the chicken and buffalo sauce to a pan. Cook for 2-3 minutes. Season with salt.

4. Divide the chicken onto lettuce leaves. Top with cheese. Roll up and serve

- **1 pound** chicken tender

- **8** large romaine lettuce leave

- **1 cup** fat free low-sodium chicken broth

- **3/4 cup** beer

- **3 tablespoons** buffalo wing sauce

- **1/2 cup** low-fat crumbled blue cheese

- salt and pepper to taste

CALORIES	CARBS	SUGAR	FAT	PROTEIN	SODIUM
92	2.0	1.0	2.1	13.1	285
KCAL	GRAMS	GRAMS	GRAMS	GRAMS	MILLIGRAMS

SEARED TANDOORI TOFU

 SERVES
5

 PREP TIME
5
MINUTES

 COOK TIME
10
MINUTES

- **1** 14-ounce **block** extra firm tofu, sliced into 1/2-inch slices

- **1 tablespoon** cayenne pepper

- **1 tablespoon** cumin

- **1 tablespoon** turmeric

- **1 tablespoon** smoked paprika

- **1/2 teaspoon** salt

- **1/2 teaspoon** black pepper

- Nonstick Cooking Spray

1. In a small bowl, mix all spices and seasoning together.

2. Spray a skillet. Heat on medium. Coat one side of the tofu and place the tofu face down. Sear both side until golden brown, around 2-3 minutes each side.

CALORIES	CARBS	SUGAR	FAT	PROTEIN	SODIUM
95	3.2	0.1	4.2	7.8	239
KCAL	GRAMS	GRAMS	GRAMS	GRAMS	MILLIGRAMS

ITALIAN PORTOBELLO BAKE

SERVES
12

PREP TIME
15
MINUTES

COOK TIME
15
MINUTES

1. Preheat the oven to 400°F.

2. Spray a large skillet, sauté mushrooms until fragrant. Season with salt and pepper. Transfer to a baking dish.

3. In a medium bowl, Mix tomatoes with all herbs. Season with salt and pepper.

4. Spread the tomato mixture on the mushrooms. Top with cheese. Bake for 20-25 minutes.

- **1 pound** Portobello Mushroom, gill removed and thinly sliced

- 1 14.5-ounce **can** crushed tomatoes

- **1 cup** fat-free parmesan cheese

- **1 cup** fat-free cheddar cheese

- **2 tablespoons** chopped fresh parsley

- **2 tablespoons** chopped fresh basil

- **1 teaspoon** dried oregano

- salt and pepper to taste

- Nonstick Cooking Spray

CALORIES	CARBS	SUGAR	FAT	PROTEIN	SODIUM
105	**14.2**	**1.2**	**1.3**	**11.6**	**393**
KCAL	GRAMS	GRAMS	GRAMS	GRAMS	MILLIGRAMS

BAKED GARLIC TOFU

 SERVES
4

 PREP TIME
10
MINUTES

 COOK TIME
40
MINUTES

- 1 14-ounce **block** firm tofu, diced

- **4 cloves** garlic, minced

- **2 tablespoons** low-sodium soy sauce

- **1 tablespoon** cornstarch

- **2 teaspoons** stevia

- **1 teaspoon** sriracha sauce

- **1 teaspoon** onion powder

1. Preheat the oven to 400°F. Bake the tofu for 35-40 minutes until golden. Flipping once.

2. Spray a sauce pan, sauté garlic until fragrant. Add soy sauce, onion powder, stevia and sriracha sauce.

3. Dissolve the cornstarch in a few tablespoons of water. Slowly stir in the cornstarch mixture. Cook until sauce thickens.

CALORIES	CARBS	SUGAR	FAT	PROTEIN	SODIUM
102	6.6	0.3	4.7	8.9	325
KCAL	GRAMS	GRAMS	GRAMS	GRAMS	MILLIGRAMS

Cooking Information Summary

Method: B-Baking   BR-Braising   G-Grilling   PF-Pan Fry   SF-Stir Fry

Recipe Name	Time (min)	Method	No. of Ingredients	No. of condiments/ spice/herbs	Dairy Free?
Beef and Vegetables Stir Fry	25	SF	6	4	Yes
Thai Ground Beef	30	BR	4	7	Yes
Spicy Beef with Bok Choy	35	SF	3	4	Yes
Beef Stuffed Bell Pepper	40	B	7	5	
Salisbury Steak with Mushroom Sauce	40	BR	8	0	Yes
Mexican Beef Skillet	45	BR	5	4	Yes
Indian Beef Curry	50	BR	6	5	
Skinny Enchiladas	55	B	6	2	
Beef Chili	70	BR	4	6	Yes
Cheese-stuffed Meatloaf	80	B	5	0	
Italian Parmesan Meatballs	90	B	4	3	
Cabbage and Beef Bake	95	B	9	0	
Beer Braised Beef	185	BR	3	3	Yes
Sichuan Spicy Beef Stew	135	BR	2	12	Yes
Mongolian Beef Skewer	490	G	1	6	Yes
Chicken and Sugar Snap Pea Stir Fry	25	SF	3	2	Yes
lemon Thyme Chicken	35	BR	3	2	Yes
Pepper stuffed Cajun chicken	35	B	4	1	

Recipe Name	Time (min)	Method	No. of Ingredients	No. of condiments/ spice/herbs	Dairy Free?
Spinach Feta Chicken Roll	35	B	5	3	
Creamy Salsa Chicken	40	B	3	1	
Yogurt Chicken Parmesan	55	B	3	1	
Hungarian Chicken Paprikash	60	BR	5	2	
Rosemary Braised Chicken	60	B	3	2	Yes
Indonesian Coconut Chicken Opor	65	BR	4	7	Yes
Italian Stuffed Chicken Breast	65	B	4	3	
White Bean and Chicken Chili	65	BR	4	6	Yes
Northern Italian Chicken Stew	70	BR	5	5	Yes
Mustard and wine braised chicken	70	BR	3	4	Yes
Yakitori Chicken	490	G	4	3	Yes
Tuna Poke	10	/	2	3	Yes
Broiled Curry Salmon	20	G	1	3	Yes
Portobello Tuna Melt	25	B	7	1	
Buffalo Ranch Salmon	25	B	2	2	Yes
Lemon Glazed Salmon	25	BR	5	2	Yes
Smoked Salmon Scramble	25	SF	4	1	Yes
Tilapia Tomato Alfredo	25	BR	5	2	
Spicy Halibut Parmesan	25	B	3	2	
Asian Salmon Meatballs	30	B	4	2	Yes
Spicy Peanut Salmon Burger	30	B	6	2	

Recipe Name	Time (min)	Method	No. of Ingredients	No. of condiments/ spice/herbs	Dairy Free?
Asian Ginger catfish	35	BR	4	4	Yes
Cheesy Tuna Mini Casserole	40	B	6	1	
Mediterranean White Fish	45	BR	5	5	
Garlic Herb Tuna Steak	50	G	2	2	Yes
Spicy Tuna Cakes	60	B	4	3	Yes
Balsamic Pork tenderloin	25	BR	5	1	Yes
Pork and Broccoli Stir Fry	25	SF	4	3	Yes
Pork Chop in Mushroom Sauce	50	BR	5	1	
Pork Chop in Creamy Onion sauce	50	BR	4	2	
Pork Stroganoff	50	BR	6	6	
Vinegar Mustard Glazed Ham Loaf	100	B	5	3	
Garlic Lemon Scallops	15	BR	4	2	Yes
Scallops in Jalapeno Whisky Cream Sauce	15	BR	4	3	
Lowcountry Shrimps	20	BR	3	2	Yes
Cheesy Onion Scallops	20	BR	5	3	
Shrimp à la Grecque	25	BR	4	3	
Crab Imperial	30	B	6	5	
Steamed Clams in Garlic Wine Sauce	35	BR	3	2	
Mussels in Marinara Sauce	40	BR	5	2	
Creamy Cajun Shrimps	40	B	5	3	
Maryland Crab Cake	75	B	3	4	

Recipe Name	Time (min)	Method	No. of Ingredients	No. of condiments/ spice/herbs	Dairy Free?
Grilled Tomato Basil Marinated Shrimp	135	G	2	5	Yes
Grilled Lemon Ginger Shrimp	135	G	2	4	Yes
Taco Salad	25	SF	6	2	
Asian Lettuce Wrap	35	SF	5	7	Yes
Shrimp Salad Stuffed tomatoes	35	/	4	3	
Sloppy Joe Lettuce Wrap	50	BR	5	3	Yes
Garden Salad with lemon chicken and Feta	60	PF	5	2	
Buffalo Chicken Lettuce Wrap	70	BR	5	1	
Seared Tandoori Tofu	15	PF	1	4	Yes
Italian Portobello Bake	30	B	3	3	
Baked Garlic Tofu	50	B	3	4	Yes

Nutrition Information Summary

Recipe Name	Calories (kCal)	Carbs (g)	Sugar (g)	Fat (g)	Protein (g)	Sodium (mg)
Beef and Vegetables Stir Fry	99	4.6	1.9	2.6	13.4	337
Thai Ground Beef	106	4.1	2.1	3.9	13.0	270
Spicy Beef with Bok Choy	114	5.7	1.6	2.6	13.5	469
Beef Stuffed Bell Pepper	118	7.7	3.6	3.2	15.6	471
Salisbury Steak with Mushroom Sauce	120	5.0	0.9	2.9	17.0	566
Mexican Beef Skillet	102	4.4	1.9	2.7	13.2	339
Indian Beef Curry	113	6.4	2.9	3.3	15.0	316
Skinny Enchiladas	149	7.5	0.6	4.3	19.9	495
Beef Chili	147	14.6	3.7	3.3	15.7	227
Cheese-stuffed Meatloaf	83	3.6	0.5	1.6	13.7	412
Italian Parmesan Meatballs	116	6.7	1.9	3.4	14.7	454
Cabbage and Beef Bake	131	9.0	4.8	3.1	17.6	313
Beer Braised Beef	96	3.6	0.8	2.0	13.0	247
Sichuan Spicy Beef Stew	84	2.4	0.7	2.0	13.0	102
Mongolian Beef Skewer	90	1.8	1.0	2.6	12.3	210
Chicken and Sugar Snap Pea Stir Fry	59	1.7	0.6	0.3	11.5	118
Lemon Thyme Chicken	55	1.0	0.2	0.2	11.3	56
Pepper stuffed Cajun chicken	91	4.0	1.6	0.6	16.3	522
Spinach Feta Chicken Roll	83	2.1	0.8	0.6	15.0	328
Creamy Salsa Chicken	92	5.5	4.0	0.2	12.0	296
Yogurt Chicken Parmesan	88	5.6	1.4	1.2	13.4	463
Hungarian Chicken Paprikash	72	3.7	1.9	0.4	12.2	80

Recipe Name	Calories (kCal)	Carbs (g)	Sugar (g)	Fat (g)	Protein (g)	Sodium (mg)
Rosemary Braised Chicken	81	1.2	0.5	0.3	11.0	57
Indonesian Coconut Chicken Opor	136	9.0	1.1	4.1	15.5	226
Italian Stuffed Chicken Breast	104	5.5	1.7	1.0	16.9	327
White Bean and Chicken Chili	115	12.0	1.7	0.6	15.2	322
Northern Italian Chicken Stew	77	4.8	2.4	0.3	11.9	145
Mustard and wine braised chicken	71	1.6	0.6	0.3	11.4	105
Yakitori Chicken	64	1.1	0.2	0.3	11.6	343
Tuna Poke	91	1.0	0.0	2.4	14.7	310
Broiled Curry Salmon	80	0.9	0.0	0.9	18.2	256
Portobello Tuna Melt	137	14.8	3.7	1.8	17.5	620
Buffalo Ranch Salmon	95	2.6	0.4	1.6	18.4	469
Lemon Glazed Salmon	83	1.8	0.2	0.8	18.7	132
Smoked Salmon Scramble	97	1.4	0.4	3.9	13.1	320
Tilapia Tomato Alfredo	84	5.8	1.8	2.1	11.3	324
Spicy Halibut Parmesan	68	3.8	0.3	0.5	12.5	270
Asian Salmon Meatballs	99	5.6	0.5	2.5	14.2	296
Spicy Peanut Salmon Burger	120	7.0	0.9	3.4	16.1	477
Asian Ginger catfish	123	3.5	1.2	1.0	12.3	518
Cheesy Tuna Mini Casserole	148	12.0	4.2	3.5	18.0	670
Mediterranean White Fish	98	3.8	1.8	1.3	14.8	340
Garlic Herb Tuna Steak	95	1.3	0.2	0.8	19.7	173
Spicy Tuna Cakes	85	4.3	0.1	3.8	8.7	312
Balsamic Pork tenderloin	77	2.7	0.8	1.4	15.0	550
Pork and Broccoli Stir Fry	78	6.0	1.3	1.2	13.0	364
Pork Chop in Mushroom Sauce	107	6.0	0.9	3.1	13.1	521
Pork Chop in Creamy Onion sauce	95	5.5	2.8	2.4	13.6	153

Recipe Name	Calories (kCal)	Carbs (g)	Sugar (g)	Fat (g)	Protein (g)	Sodium (mg)
Pork Stroganoff	93	7.3	2.7	1.5	13.6	448
Vinegar Mustard Glazed Ham Loaf	146	9.6	4.3	4.7	17.3	755
Garlic Lemon Scallops	72	5.2	0.2	0.5	11.7	450
Scallops in Jalapeno Whisky Cream Sauce	96	7.1	1.7	0.9	12.4	623
Lowcountry Shrimps	75	1.2	0.4	1.6	13.5	448
Cheesy Onion Scallops	94	6.0	0.3	0.5	12.1	460
Shrimp à la Grecque	97	4.3	1.7	0.9	14.1	507
Crab Imperial	76	10.8	4.9	0.6	7.4	423
Steamed Clams in Garlic Wine Sauce	168	5.7	0.1	3.6	18.9	111
Mussels in Marinara Sauce	174	8.1	1.3	4.9	16.9	410
Creamy Cajun Shrimps	69	1.2	0.4	1.3	12.7	485
Maryland Crab Cake	69	4.1	0.6	0.7	11.5	346
Grilled Tomato Basil Marinated Shrimp	77	0.9	0.5	2.6	12.2	361
Grilled Lemon Ginger Shrimp	66	1.9	0.3	1.0	12.4	345
Taco Salad	134	7.6	2.7	.2.4	21.8	376
Asian Lettuce Wrap	121	9.0	3.5	4.1	13.0	351
Shrimp Salad Stuffed tomatoes	80	4.5	2.8	1.3	12.9	309
Sloppy Joe Lettuce Wrap	82	3.6	1.6	2.2	12.8	155
Garden Salad with lemon chicken and Feta	111	8.5	3.1	2.9	12.9	475
Buffalo Chicken Lettuce Wrap	92	2.0	1.0	2.1	13.1	285
Seared Tandoori Tofu	95	3.2	0.1	4.2	7.8	239
Italian Portobello Bake	105	14.2	1.2	1.3	11.6	393
Baked Garlic Tofu	102	6.6	0.3	4.7	8.9	325

BEEF AND EGGPLANT CASSEROLE

 SERVES 16

 PREP TIME 10 MINUTES

 COOK TIME 5 HOURS

- **2 pounds** 95/5 ground beef
- **2 cups** cubed eggplant
- **1** 28-ounce **can** diced tomatoes, drained
- **2 cups** tomato sauce
- **2 cups** fat-free shredded mozzarella cheese
- **2 teaspoons** mustard
- **2 teaspoons** Worcestershire sauce
- **1 teaspoon** dried oregano
- **1 teaspoon** salt
- **1/2 teaspoon** pepper

1. Sprinkle cut eggplant with salt and let sit in a colander for about 30 minutes.

2. In a large bowl, combine beef, Worcestershire sauce, mustard, salt and pepper. Spread the mixture on the bottom of the slow cooker.

3. Spread eggplant on top. Spread tomatoes and tomato sauce. Top with mozzarella and sprinkle with oregano.

4. Cover and cook on low for 4-5 hours

CALORIES	CARBS	SUGAR	FAT	PROTEIN	SODIUM
117	5.4	2.6	3.1	17.4	546
KCAL	GRAMS	GRAMS	GRAMS	GRAMS	MILLIGRAMS

LOW CARB PIZZA

 SERVES 16

 PREP TIME 15 **MINUTES**

 COOK TIME 6 **HOURS**

1. Brown the beef. Transfer to a large bowl. Combine with onion and sauce.

2. Spray the slow cooker. Spread half of the meat mixture on the bottom. Lay half of the spinach on top. Lay 1/2 of the mushrooms, bell peppers and pepperoni then top with cheese. Repeat the layers with mozzarella on top.

3. Cook on low for 5-6 hours.

- **1 1/2 pounds** 95/5 ground beef
- **2 cups** no-sugar-added pasta sauce
- **3 cups** baby spinach
- **2 cups** sliced mushrooms
- **1/2 cup** sliced bell peppers
- **1/2 cup** chopped onion
- **16 slices** low fat pepperoni
- **3 cups** fat-free shredded mozzarella
- Nonstick Cooking Spray

CALORIES	CARBS	SUGAR	FAT	PROTEIN	SODIUM
113	4.6	1.3	2.7	17.1	512
KCAL	GRAMS	GRAMS	GRAMS	GRAMS	MILLIGRAMS

EASY SWISS STEAK

 SERVES
12

 PREP TIME
10
MINUTES

 COOK TIME
7
HOURS

- **1 1/2 pounds** lean top round roast

- **1** 28-ounce **can** crushed tomatoes, with juice

- **1** medium onion, sliced

- **1 envelop** onion soup mix

- **1 teaspoon** dried oregano

- **1/2 teaspoon** salt

- **1/2 teaspoon** pepper

1. In a small bowl mix together oregano, salt and pepper. Rub the seasoning on the roast.

2. Brown the roast on all side. Transfer to slow cooker. Top with the remaining ingredients

3. Cook on low for 7-8 hours.

CALORIES	CARBS	SUGAR	FAT	PROTEIN	SODIUM
108	7.0	2.4	3.0	13.3	307
KCAL	GRAMS	GRAMS	GRAMS	GRAMS	MILLIGRAMS

ORANGE BEEF

SERVES
12

PREP TIME
15
MINUTES

COOK TIME
7
HOURS

1. Add all ingredients slow cooker.

2. Cool on low for 7-8 hours or until meat is tender.

- **1 1/2 pounds** lean sirloin steak, cut into 1/4-inch slices

- **2 1/2 cups** sliced mushrooms

- **1** medium onion, diced

- **2 cloves** garlic, minced

- **1/2 cup** fresh orange juice

- **1/2 cup** low-sodium soy sauce

- **1/4 cup** apple cider vinegar

- **2 tablespoons** stevia

- **1 tablespoon** grated fresh ginger

- **1 tablespoon** sesame oil

CALORIES	CARBS	SUGAR	FAT	PROTEIN	SODIUM
109	4.2	0.9	3.7	13.7	569
KCAL	GRAMS	GRAMS	GRAMS	GRAMS	MILLIGRAMS

CHINESE DAIKON BEEF STEW

 SERVES
12

 PREP TIME
15
MINUTES

 COOK TIME
8
HOURS

- **2 pounds** lean top round roast, cut into 1.5-inch cubes

- **1 pound** Daikon Radish, halved lengthwise and cut into 1.5-inch pieces

- **3 cloves** garlic, minced

- **2 tablespoons** grated fresh ginger

- **2** star anise

- **1** bay leave

- **2 tablespoons** Oyster Sauce

- **2 tablespoons** cooking wine

- **1 tablespoon** Hoisin Sauce

- **1 tablespoon** low-sodium soy sauce

- salt to taste

1. Spray a skillet, Brown the beef then transfer to slow cooker.

2. Sauté the garlic and ginger until fragrant. Transfer to slow cooker.

3. Add the remaining ingredients except Daikon and mix well.

4. Cover and cook on low for 7-8 hours. Add the Daikon in the last 1 hour. Add salt to taste.

CALORIES	CARBS	SUGAR	FAT	PROTEIN	SODIUM
107	3.3	1.6	2.8	17.4	218
KCAL	GRAMS	GRAMS	GRAMS	GRAMS	MILLIGRAMS

ASIAN BRAISED BEEF

 SERVES
16

 PREP TIME
15
MINUTES

 COOK TIME
6
HOURS

1. In a small bowl mix together flour, salt and pepper. Coat the beef with the mixture.

2. Spray a skillet, Brown the beef then transfer to slow cooker.

3. Sauté the garlic and ginger until fragrant. Transfer to the slow cooker.

4. Add all the remaining ingredients and stir well.

5. Cover and cook on low for 7-8 hours

- **2 pounds** lean top round roast, cut into 1.5-inch cubes
- **2 cloves** garlic, minced
- **1** green onion, thinly sliced
- **1 tablespoon** grated fresh ginger
- **1/2 stalk** lemongrass, pounded
- **1/2 cup** fat-free low-sodium chicken broth
- **1/2 cup** white rice vinegar
- **1/4 cup** hoisin sauce
- **1/4 cup** Stevia
- **1 tablespoon** Sriracha Sauce
- **1 tablespoon** whole wheat flour
- **1 teaspoon** crushed red pepper flakes
- **1/2 teaspoon** salt
- **1/4 teaspoon** ground black pepper
- Nonstick Cooking Spray

CALORIES	CARBS	SUGAR	FAT	PROTEIN	SODIUM
114	4.3	1.8	2.9	17.1	248
KCAL	GRAMS	GRAMS	GRAMS	GRAMS	MILLIGRAMS

TRADITIONAL TEXAS CHILI

 SERVES
16

 PREP TIME
20
MINUTES

 COOK TIME
8
HOURS

- **2 pounds** lean top round roast, cubed

- **2** 14-ounce **cans** diced tomatoes, with juice

- **1** 4-ounce **can** chopped green chili, drained

- **1** medium onion, minced

- **4 cloves** garlic, minced

- **2** jalapeño peppers, minced

- **3 cups** fat-free low sodium beef broth

- **3 tablespoons** chili powder

- **2 tablespoons** whole wheat flour

- **1 tablespoon** ground cumin

- **1 teaspoon** crushed red pepper

- **1 teaspoon** dried oregano

- **1 teaspoon** salt

1. In a small bowl mix together flour, salt and pepper. Coat the beef with the mixture.

2. Spray a skillet, Brown the beef then transfer to slow cooker.

3. Sauté the garlic, onion, green chili and jalapeño peppers until fragrant. Transfer to the slow cooker.

4. Add all the remaining ingredients and stir well.

5. Cover and cook on low for 7-8 hours

CALORIES	CARBS	SUGAR	FAT	PROTEIN	SODIUM
94	5.0	1.1	2.3	14.5	359
KCAL	GRAMS	GRAMS	GRAMS	GRAMS	MILLIGRAMS

RICELESS CABBAGE ROLL

 SERVES
8

 PREP TIME
15
MINUTES

 COOK TIME
8
HOURS

1. Steam the cauliflower for 5-6 minutes. Use a food processor to break into rice-like texture.

2. Blanch the cabbage leaves for 2 minutes. Set aside.

3. In a large bowl, mix together beef, cauliflower, egg, milk, salt and pepper. Divide the mixture into 12 portions and spoon onto the cabbage leave. Roll up and put in slow cooker.

4. In a small bowl, mix together tomato sauce, stevia, lemon juice and Worcestershire sauce. Spread the sauce on the rolls.

5. Cover and cook on low for 7-8 hours

- **1 pound** 95/5 ground beef
- **12** cabbage leaves
- **1 cup** chopped cauliflower
- **1** egg, beaten
- **1 cup** tomato sauce
- **1/4 cup** skim milk
- **1/4 cup** chopped onion
- **1 tablespoon** lemon juice
- **1 teaspoon** Worcestershire Sauce
- **1/2 teaspoon** salt
- **1/2 teaspoon** ground black pepper
- **1/2 teaspoon** stevia

CALORIES	CARBS	SUGAR	FAT	PROTEIN	SODIUM
111	6.1	3.4	3.7	14.2	360
KCAL	GRAMS	GRAMS	GRAMS	GRAMS	MILLIGRAMS

CLASSIC BEEF STEW

SERVES
16

PREP TIME
10
MINUTES

COOK TIME
8.5
HOURS

- **2 pounds** lean top round roast, cubed

- **6 stalks** celery, roughly chopped

- **3** medium carrots, roughly chopped

- **1** medium onion, roughly chopped

- **2 cups** fat-free low sodium beef broth

- **2 tablespoons** corn starch

- **3** bay leaves

- **1 teaspoon** dried thyme

- **1 teaspoon** chili powder

- **1 teaspoon** salt

1. Add all ingredients except cornstarch in slow cooker.

2. Cover and cook on low for 7-8 hours.

3. Dissolve cornstarch in a few tablespoons of water. Slowly stir in the soup. Cook on high for 30 minutes.

CALORIES	CARBS	SUGAR	FAT	PROTEIN	SODIUM
113	5.3	1.2	2.7	17.3	291
KCAL	GRAMS	GRAMS	GRAMS	GRAMS	MILLIGRAMS

SHREDDED BEEF PORTOBELLO OPEN SANDWICH

 SERVES 8

 PREP TIME 15 MINUTES

 COOK TIME 8.5 HOURS

1. In a small bowl, mix all spices and seasoning. Rub them on the roast evenly.

2. Brown the roast on all sides. Transfer to slow cooker. Add vinegar and water.

3. Cover and cook on low for 7-8 hours.

4. Preheat the broiler. Broil the mushroom for 5 minutes. Set aside

5. Remove the meat and shred the meat.

6. Skim off the fat on the sauce and stir in mustard. Return meat and mix well. Spoon the meat mixture on the mushroom and serve.

- **1 1/2 pounds** lean top round roast
- **6** large Portobello mushrooms
- **1/3 cup** water
- **1 tablespoon** Dijon mustard
- **1/2 tablespoon** red wine vinegar
- **1/2 teaspoon** dried basil
- **1/2 teaspoon** dried oregano
- **1/2 teaspoon** crushed rosemary
- **1/2 teaspoon** garlic powder
- **1/2 teaspoon** onion powder
- **1/2 teaspoon** salt
- **1/4 teaspoon** ground black pepper
- Nonstick Cooking Spray

CALORIES	CARBS	SUGAR	FAT	PROTEIN	SODIUM
108	0.9	0.4	3.1	19.3	237
KCAL	GRAMS	GRAMS	GRAMS	GRAMS	MILLIGRAMS

BROCCOLI AND BEEF

 SERVES
16

 PREP TIME
15
MINUTES

 COOK TIME
8.5
HOURS

- **1 1/2 pounds** lean sirloin steak, cut into 1/4-inch slices

- **1 1/2 pounds** broccoli floret

- **2 cloves** garlic

- **1** beef bouillon cube

- **1 cup** warm water

- **1/2 cup** low sodium soy sauce

- **2 tablespoons** stevia

- **2 tablespoons** corn starch

1. Dissolve the beef bouillon cube in warm water. Stir in soy sauce, stevia and garlic.

2. Add beef and sauce mixture to slow cooker. Cover and cook on low for 6-8 hours.

3. Dissolve cornstarch in a few tablespoons of water. Stir in. Cover and cook on high for 30 minutes. Meanwhile steam the broccoli until tender.

4. Toss in the broccoli. Mix well and serve.

CALORIES	CARBS	SUGAR	FAT	PROTEIN	SODIUM
101	5.7	1.0	2.7	14.0	321
KCAL	GRAMS	GRAMS	GRAMS	GRAMS	MILLIGRAMS

BEEF IN MUSHROOM SAUCE

 SERVES
8

 PREP TIME
25
MINUTES

 COOK TIME
8.5
HOURS

1. Add mushrooms to slow cooker.

2. Season the beef with salt and pepper. Brown the beef. Transfer to slow cooker. Add wine, broth and Worcestershire sauce.

3. Cover and cook on low for 7-8 hours.

4. Dissolve cornstarch in a few tablespoons of cool water. Stir in. Cover and cook on high for 30 minutes.

- **1 1/2 pounds** lean sirloin steak, cubed

- **3 cups** sliced mushrooms

- **2 cups** fat-free ow sodium beef broth

- **1/3 cup** dry red wine

- **2 tablespoons** corn starch

- **1 tablespoon** Worcestershire sauce

- **1/2 teaspoon** salt

- **1/4 teaspoon** pepper

- Nonstick Cooking spray

CALORIES	CARBS	SUGAR	FAT	PROTEIN	SODIUM
96	2.7	0.1	2.5	13.4	336
KCAL	GRAMS	GRAMS	GRAMS	GRAMS	MILLIGRAMS

ROUND ROAST IN APPLE AND ONION SAUCE

 SERVES
12

 PREP TIME
30
MINUTES

 COOK TIME
8.5
HOURS

- **2 pounds** lean top round roast
- **1 large** onion, sliced
- **1 large** apple, quartered
- **1 cup** of water
- **2 tablespoons** cornstarch
- **1 teaspoon** salt
- **1/2 teaspoon** low-sodium soy sauce
- **1/2 teaspoon** Worcestershire Sauce
- **1/4 teaspoon** garlic powder
- Non-stick Cooking Spray

1. Rub the roast with salt and pepper. Brown the roast on all side. Transfer to slow cooker.

2. Add water, soy sauce, Worcestershire sauce and garlic powder. Mix well and top with onion and apple.

3. Cover and Cook on low for 7-8 hours.

4. Set aside the roast and onion. Discard the apple. Transfer the sauce to a saucepan. Bring to a boil. Reduce to low heat and simmer for 15 minutes.

5. Dissolve cornstarch in a with tablespoons of water. Slowly stir in the sauce and cook until thickened. Serve over sliced roast.

CALORIES	CARBS	SUGAR	FAT	PROTEIN	SODIUM
110	5.0	2.4	2.7	16.9	260
KCAL	GRAMS	GRAMS	GRAMS	GRAMS	MILLIGRAMS

CUBAN SHREDDED BEEF

 SERVES
12

 PREP TIME
30
MINUTES

 COOK TIME
10
HOURS

1. In a small bowl mix together oregano, cumin, salt and pepper. Rub the seasoning on the roast.

2. Brown the roast on all side. Transfer to slow cooker.

3. Sauté the bell peppers, garlic and onion until fragrant. Add crushed tomatoes and simmer for 4 minutes. Transfer to slow cooker.

4. Cover and cook on low for 10 hours. Shred the meat and serve with   pimiento-stuffed green olives

- **2 pounds** lean top round roast
- 1 large onion, roughly chopped
- 2 medium bell peppers, roughly chopped
- **2 cups** crushed tomatoes
- **16** pimiento-stuffed green olives
- **1 teaspoon** dried oregano
- **1 teaspoon** ground cumin
- **1 teaspoon** salt
- **1/2 teaspoon** pepper
- Nonstick Cooking Spray

CALORIES	CARBS	SUGAR	FAT	PROTEIN	SODIUM
122	5.6	2.3	3.0	17.7	380
KCAL	GRAMS	GRAMS	GRAMS	GRAMS	MILLIGRAMS

SPICY BEEF ROAST

 SERVES
12

 PREP TIME
15
MINUTES

 COOK TIME
10.5
HOURS

- **2 pounds** lean top round roast
- **2 cups** water
- **1 envelop** onion soup mix
- **2 cloves** garlic, minced
- **1/4 cup** low sugar low salt ketchup
- **2 tablespoons** Worcestershire Sauce
- **2 tablespoons** cornstarch
- **1/2 teaspoon** salt
- **1/4 teaspoon** ground black pepper

1. In a small bowl mix together salt and pepper. Rub the seasoning on the roast.

2. Brown the roast on all side. Transfer to slow cooker. Top with the remaining ingredients except corn starch

3. Cook on low for 9-10 hours.

4. Dissolve the cornstarch in a few tablespoons of water. Stir in the sauce. Cook on high for 30 minutes. Slice the beef and serve with gravy.

CALORIES	CARBS	SUGAR	FAT	PROTEIN	SODIUM
102	2.7	0.6	2.7	16.8	217
KCAL	GRAMS	GRAMS	GRAMS	GRAMS	MILLIGRAMS

BUFFALO RANCH CHICKEN

 SERVES
8

 PREP TIME
5
MINUTES

 COOK TIME
6
HOURS

1. Add Chicken to the slow cooker.

2. In a small bowl, combine broth, buffalo and ranch seasoning. Pour over the chicken.

3. Cover and cook on low for 5-6 hours.

4. Top with crumbled blue cheese and serve.

- **1 1/2 pounds** chicken tender
- **1/2 cup** fat-free low-sodium chicken broth
- **1/2 cup** buffalo sauce
- **1 tablespoon** ranch seasoning
- **1/4 cup** low-fat blue cheese crumble

CALORIES	CARBS	SUGAR	FAT	PROTEIN	SODIUM
109	0.3	0.1	3.4	17.4	481
KCAL	GRAMS	GRAMS	GRAMS	GRAMS	MILLIGRAMS

CREAMY CHICKEN WITH BLACK BEAN

 SERVES
12

 PREP TIME
5
MINUTES

 COOK TIME
6
HOURS

- **1 1/2 pounds** chicken tender
- **1** 15-ounce **can** black beans, rinsed and drained
- **2 cups** salsa
- **8 ounces** fat-free cream cheese

1. Add chicken, beans and salsa to slow cooker.

2. Cook on low for 5-6 hours.

3. Shred the chicken. Return to the pot. Stir in cream cheese. Let it sit for 15 minutes before serving.

CALORIES	CARBS	SUGAR	FAT	PROTEIN	SODIUM
116	10.1	2.7	0.8	16.8	562
KCAL	GRAMS	GRAMS	GRAMS	GRAMS	MILLIGRAMS

CREAMY MEXICAN CHICKEN

 SERVES 12

 PREP TIME 5 MINUTES

 COOK TIME 6 HOURS

1. Add all ingredients in the slow cooker. Stir to mix well.

2. Cover and cook on low for 5-6 hours.

- **2 pounds** chicken tender
- 1 14.5-ounce **can** diced tomatoes and green chilies
- **1 cup** fat-free sour cream
- **1/2 cup** fat-free low sodium chicken broth
- **1 package** Taco seasoning

CALORIES	CARBS	SUGAR	FAT	PROTEIN	SODIUM
89	3.8	2.2	0.3	16.5	251
KCAL	GRAMS	GRAMS	GRAMS	GRAMS	MILLIGRAMS

CHICKEN FAJITA SOUP

 SERVES
8

 PREP TIME
5
MINUTES

 COOK TIME
6
HOURS

- **1 1/2 pounds** chicken tender, cut into bite size

- **1 14.5-ounce can** diced tomatoes

- **1** medium onion, diced

- **1** medium bell pepper, diced

- **1 cup** sliced mushrooms

- **2 cloves** garlic, minced

- **3 1/2 cups** fat-free low sodium chicken broth

- **1 package** Taco seasoning

- **2 tablespoons** chopped fresh cilantro

- salt and pepper to taste

1. Add all ingredients except cilantro in the slow cooker. Stir to mix well.

2. Cover and cook on low for 5-6 hours. Sprinkle with cilantro and serve

CALORIES	CARBS	SUGAR	FAT	PROTEIN	SODIUM
105	5.7	1.3	0.4	18.8	305
KCAL	GRAMS	GRAMS	GRAMS	GRAMS	MILLIGRAMS

VINEGAR SHREDDED CHICKEN

 SERVES 4

 PREP TIME 10 MINUTES

 COOK TIME 6 HOURS

1. Place the chicken in the slow cooker.

2. In a small bowl, combine the remaining ingredients and pour over chicken.

3. Cover and cook on low for 6 hours. Shred the chicken and return to the slow cooker. Let it sit for 15 minutes before serving.

- **1 pound** boneless skinless chicken breast

- **2 cups** water

- **1 cup** white vinegar

- **2 tablespoons** stevia

- **1 tablespoon** low-sodium chicken base

- **1 teaspoon** crushed red pepper flakes

- **3/4 teaspoon** salt

CALORIES	CARBS	SUGAR	FAT	PROTEIN	SODIUM
116	2.8	1.2	0.8	23.6	589
KCAL	GRAMS	GRAMS	GRAMS	GRAMS	MILLIGRAMS

BARBEQUE CHICKEN

 SERVES
6

 PREP TIME
10
MINUTES

 COOK TIME
6
HOURS

- **1 pound** chicken tender

- **1/3 cup** low-sugar low salt ketchup

- **1/4 cup** fresh orange juice

- **2 tablespoons** water

- **2 tablespoons** red wine vinegar

- **1 tablespoon** stevia, preferably brown sugar blend

- **1 tablespoon** olive oil

- **1 tablespoon** chopped fresh parsley

- **1 teaspoon** Worcestershire sauce

- **1/2 teaspoon** salt

- **1/4 teaspoon** pepper

1. Place the chicken in the slow cooker.

2. In a small bowl, combine the remaining ingredients and pour over chicken.

3. Cover and cook on low for 6 hours. Shred the chicken and return to the slow cooker. Let it sit for 15 minutes before serving.

CALORIES	CARBS	SUGAR	FAT	PROTEIN	SODIUM
98	2.9	1.8	2.6	14.7	273
KCAL	GRAMS	GRAMS	GRAMS	GRAMS	MILLIGRAMS

SWEET AND SOUR CHICKEN

 SERVES 6

 PREP TIME 10 MINUTES

 COOK TIME 6 HOURS

1. Place the chicken in the slow cooker.

2. In a small bowl, combine the remaining ingredients except cornstarch and pour over chicken.

3. Cover and cook on low for 5.5 hours.

4. Dissolve the cornstarch in a few tablespoons of water. Stir in. Cover and cook on high for 30 minutes.

- **1 pound** chicken breast, cut into 2-inch pieces

- **2 cloves** garlic, minced

- **1/4 cup** apple cider vinegar

- **2 tablespoons** stevia, preferably brown sugar blend

- **2 tablespoons** low-sugar low salt ketchup

- **2 tablespoons** low-sodium soy sauce

- **2 tablespoons** water

- **1 tablespoons** olive oil

- **1/4 teaspoon** pepper

CALORIES	CARBS	SUGAR	FAT	PROTEIN	SODIUM
103	5.1	2.4	2.6	15.1	272
KCAL	GRAMS	GRAMS	GRAMS	GRAMS	MILLIGRAMS

CREAMY PORTOBELLO CHICKEN

SERVES
6

PREP TIME
10
MINUTES

COOK TIME
6
HOURS

- **1 pound** chicken tender, cut into 2-inch pieces

- **3 cups** sliced baby Portobello mushroom

- **1** 10.5-ounce **can** 98% fat free cream of chicken soup

- salt and pepper to taste

1. Place the chicken in the slow cooker. Top with sliced mushrooms. Pour the soup over and sprinkle with salt and pepper.

2. Cover and cook on low for 5-6 hours.

CALORIES	CARBS	SUGAR	FAT	PROTEIN	SODIUM
116	7.2	1.4	1.4	17.5	663
KCAL	GRAMS	GRAMS	GRAMS	GRAMS	MILLIGRAMS

CHICKEN CACCIATORE

 SERVES
12

 PREP TIME
15
MINUTES

 COOK TIME
6
HOURS

1. Add tomato paste and broth the slow cooker and mix well.

2. In a small bowl, mix rosemary, salt and pepper. Rub them on the chicken breast evenly. Place in the slow cooker. Top with the remaining ingredients.

3. Cover and cook on low for 5-6 hours.

- **2 pounds** chicken tender
- **1** 8-ounce **can** tomato paste
- **3 cups** sliced mushrooms
- **2 cups** sliced red pepper
- **1 cup** chopped onion
- **2 cloves** garlic, minced
- **1 cup** fat-free low-sodium chicken broth
- **1 teaspoon** dried rosemary
- **1/2 teaspoon** salt
- **1/2 teaspoon** pepper

CALORIES	CARBS	SUGAR	FAT	PROTEIN	SODIUM
109	**7.7**	**3.5**	**0.4**	**17.5**	**368**
KCAL	GRAMS	GRAMS	GRAMS	GRAMS	MILLIGRAMS

CREAMY LIME CHICKEN

SERVES
12

PREP TIME
20
MINUTES

COOK TIME
6
HOURS

- **2 pounds** chicken tender

- **2 cups** fat-free low sodium chicken broth

- **1/2 cup** fat-free half-and-half

- **1/4 cup** lime juice

- **2 tablespoons** chopped fresh cilantro

- **1 tablespoon** cornstarch

- **1 tablespoon** olive oil

- **1 tablespoon** chili powder

- **1 teaspoon** cumin

- **1/2 teaspoon** paprika

- **1/2 teaspoon** salt

1. In a small bowl, mix paprika, thyme, salt and pepper. Rub them on the chicken breast evenly.Sear the chicken on both side until golden brown. Transfer to slow cooker.

2. Add lime juice and broth. Cover and cook on low for 5-6 hours. Dissolve cornstarch in a few tablespoons of water. Stir in cornstarch mixture, half-and-half and cilantro in the last 15 minutes.

CALORIES	CARBS	SUGAR	FAT	PROTEIN	SODIUM
91	2.5	0.6	1.7	15.4	209
KCAL	GRAMS	GRAMS	GRAMS	GRAMS	MILLIGRAMS

CHICKEN AND KALE SOUP

SERVES
8

PREP TIME
10
MINUTES

COOK TIME
7
HOURS

1. Place the chicken in the slow cooker. Top with garlic and onion. Pour broth over.

2. Cover and cook on low for 5-6 hours. Add carrot and kale. Cover and cook on low for 1 hour. Sprinkle with parsley and serve.

- **1 1/2 pounds** chicken tender, cut into bite size

- **1** medium onion, diced

- **4 cups** chopped kale

- **1 cup** shredded carrots

- **3 1/2 cups** fat-free low sodium chicken stock

- **2 teaspoons** chopped fresh parsley

- salt and pepper to taste

CALORIES	CARBS	SUGAR	FAT	PROTEIN	SODIUM
95	3.9	0.6	0.5	18.1	125
KCAL	GRAMS	GRAMS	GRAMS	GRAMS	MILLIGRAMS

WHITE CHICKEN CHILI

SERVES
12

PREP TIME
15
MINUTES

COOK TIME
7
HOURS

- **1 pound** chicken tender, cut into 1-inch cubes

- **2** 15.5-ounce **cans** Cannelloni beans, rinsed and drained

- **1** 4-ounce **can** chopped green chili peppers

- **2 cups** chopped onion

- **2 cloves** garlic, minced

- **3 cups** fat-free low sodium chicken broth

- **1 teaspoon** salt

- **1 teaspoon** ground cumin

- **3/4 teaspoon** dried oregano

- **1/2 teaspoon** chili powder

- **1/2 teaspoon** ground black pepper

- **1/8 teaspoon** ground cloves

1. Brown the meat. Transfer to slow cooker. Discard excess fat.

2. Add the remaining ingredients to slow cooker and mix well.

3. Cover and cook on low for 6-8 hours

CALORIES	CARBS	SUGAR	FAT	PROTEIN	SODIUM
107	**13.6**	**1.1**	**0.3**	**11.5**	**675**
KCAL	GRAMS	GRAMS	GRAMS	GRAMS	MILLIGRAMS

FIESTA CHICKEN SOUP

 SERVES
12

 PREP TIME
5
MINUTES

 COOK TIME
8
HOURS

1. Add all ingredients in slow cooker.

2. Cook on low for 6-8 hours.

- **1 pound** chicken tender, cut into 1-inch cubes
- **1 15.5-ounce can** black beans, rinsed and drained
- **1 15.5-ounce can** kidney beans, rinsed and drained
- **1 14.5-ounce can** diced tomatoes
- **1 4-ounce can** diced green chili peppers
- **2 1/2 cups** fat-free low sodium chicken broth
- **1/2 cup** chopped fresh cilantro
- **1/2 cup** chopped onion
- **2 cloves** garlic, minced
- **1** lime, juice only
- **1 tablespoon** chili powder
- **1 teaspoon** ground cumin
- **1/2 teaspoon** ground black pepper
- salt to taste

CALORIES	CARBS	SUGAR	FAT	PROTEIN	SODIUM
98	**11.0**	**1.6**	**0.7**	**12.1**	**299**
KCAL	GRAMS	GRAMS	GRAMS	GRAMS	MILLIGRAMS

SPINACH ARTICHOKE CHICKEN

 SERVES
12

 PREP TIME
5
MINUTES

 COOK TIME
8
HOURS

- **1 1/2 pounds** chicken tender

- **8 cups** chopped fresh spinach

- **1** 14-ounce **can** artichoke hearts

- **1 cup** chopped tomatoes

- **3 cloves** garlic, minced

- **1 cup** fat free low-sodium chicken broth

- **2 ounces** fat-free cream cheese

- **1/4 cup** fat-free shredded parmesan cheese

- salt and pepper to taste

1. Place the chicken and spinach in the slow cooker. Top with garlic. Pour broth over.

2. Cover and cook on low for 6-8 hours.

3. Remove and shred the chicken.

4. Add cream cheese, parmesan cheese and artichokes to the slow cooker. Stir until creamy. Return the chicken and mix well. Top with tomatoes before serving.

CALORIES	CARBS	SUGAR	FAT	PROTEIN	SODIUM
123	11.0	3.5	0.3	17.3	586
KCAL	GRAMS	GRAMS	GRAMS	GRAMS	MILLIGRAMS

GARLIC CHICKEN PARMESAN

 SERVES
16

 PREP TIME
15
MINUTES

 COOK TIME
6
HOURS

1. In a small bowl, mix all spices and seasoning except thyme. Rub them on the chicken breast evenly. Place in the slow cooker. Top with garlic and drizzle with olive oil.

2. Cover and cook on low for 6-8 hours. Sprinkle with Parmesan and serve.

- **2 pounds** chicken tender
- **4 cloves** garlic, minced
- **1 cup** fat-free grated parmesan cheese
- **1 tablespoon** olive oil
- **1 teaspoon** salt
- **1/2 teaspoon** dried thyme
- **1/2 teaspoon** dried basil
- **1/2 teaspoon** dried oregano
- **1/4 teaspoon** dried rosemary

CALORIES	CARBS	SUGAR	FAT	PROTEIN	SODIUM
99	4.4	0.0	1.5	16.1	437
KCAL	GRAMS	GRAMS	GRAMS	GRAMS	MILLIGRAMS

CURRY CHICKEN

 SERVES
8

 PREP TIME
10
MINUTES

 COOK TIME
8
HOURS

- **1 1/2 pounds** chicken tender

- **1 14-ounce can** light coconut milk

- **1 medium** onion, diced

- **3 cloves** garlic, minced

- **2 bay** leaves

- **2 tablespoons** tomato paste

- **2 tablespoons** grated fresh ginger

- **1 teaspoon** cumin

- **1 teaspoon** turmeric

- **1 teaspoon** garam masala

- **1 teaspoon** salt

1. Place the chicken in the slow cooker.

2. In a small bowl, combine the remaining ingredients and pour over chicken.

3. Cover and cook on low for 7-8 hours. Shred the chicken and return to the slow cooker. Let it sit for 15 minutes before serving.

CALORIES	CARBS	SUGAR	FAT	PROTEIN	SODIUM
125	6.5	1.7	3.0	17.1	387
KCAL	GRAMS	GRAMS	GRAMS	GRAMS	MILLIGRAMS

MEXICAN TURKEY CASSEROLE

 SERVES
16

 PREP TIME
10
MINUTES

 COOK TIME
8
HOURS

1. Brown the meat. Transfer to slow cooker. Discard excess fat.

2. Add the remaining ingredients except cheese to slow cooker and mix well.

3. Cover and cook on low for 6-8 hours.

4. Stir in half of cheese and sprinkle the rest on top. Cover and cook on high for 15 minutes.

- **1 1/2 pounds** 95/5 ground turkey
- **1** medium onion, diced
- **2** 10-ounce **cans** enchiladas sauce
- **2** 15-ounce **cans** black beans, rinsed and drained
- **1** 14.5-ounce **can** fire-roasted diced tomatoes
- **3** bell peppers, diced
- **1 cup** low-fat shredded Mexican Cheese, divided
- **2 tablespoons** chili powder
- **1 tablespoon** ground cumin
- **1 teaspoon** garlic powder

CALORIES	CARBS	SUGAR	FAT	PROTEIN	SODIUM
134	14.7	1.3	2.4	16.0	582
KCAL	GRAMS	GRAMS	GRAMS	GRAMS	MILLIGRAMS

SPICY PEPPER CHICKEN

 SERVES
6

 PREP TIME
10
MINUTES

 COOK TIME
8
HOURS

- **1 pound** chicken tender
- **2** green onions, chopped
- **1** bell pepper, diced
- **1** large chili pepper, sliced
- **1** jalapeno pepper, sliced
- **1 clove** garlic, minced
- **1/2 cup** fat-free low sodium chicken broth
- **1 tablespoon** powdered peanut butter
- **2 teaspoons** lemon juice
- **2 teaspoons** soy sauce
- **1 teaspoon** olive oil
- **1/2 teaspoon** ground ginger
- **1/4 teaspoon** fresh ground black pepper
- salt to taste

1. Place the chicken in the slow cooker. Top with all vegetables.

2. In a small bowl, combine the remaining ingredients. Pour the sauce over and sprinkle with salt and pepper.

3. Cover and cook on low for 6-8 hours.

CALORIES	CARBS	SUGAR	FAT	PROTEIN	SODIUM
94	3.7	1.3	1.4	16.3	161
KCAL	GRAMS	GRAMS	GRAMS	GRAMS	MILLIGRAMS

SIMPLE TURKEY CHILI

 SERVES
16

 PREP TIME
15
MINUTES

 COOK TIME
8
HOURS

1. Brown the meat. Transfer to slow cooker. Discard excess fat.

2. Add the remaining ingredients to slow cooker and mix well.

3. Cover and cook on low for 6-8 hours

- **1 1/2 pounds** 95/5 ground turkey

- **1** 15.5-ounce **can** kidney beans, rinsed and drained

- **1** 15-ounce **can** black beans, rinsed and drained

- **1** 14.5-ounce **can** diced tomatoes

- **1** 8-ounce **can** tomato paste

- **1 cup** tomato juice

- **1/2 cup** chopped onion

- **2 1/2 cups** water

- **2 1/2 tablespoons** chili powder

- **1 teaspoon** salt

CALORIES	CARBS	SUGAR	FAT	PROTEIN	SODIUM
109	11.5	3.2	0.8	14.9	397
KCAL	GRAMS	GRAMS	GRAMS	GRAMS	MILLIGRAMS

HONEY MUSTARD CHICKEN STEW

 SERVES
6

 PREP TIME
15
MINUTES

 COOK TIME
8
HOURS

- **1 pound** chicken tender, cut into 1-inch cubes

- **1 1/2 cups** chopped celery

- **1 1/2 cups** chopped onion

- **1/2 cup** chopped carrots

- **1 cup** fat-free low sodium chicken broth

- **2 tablespoons** Dijon mustard

- **1 tablespoon** Truvia Nectar

- **1 teaspoon** dried rosemary

1. Brown the meat. Transfer to slow cooker. Discard excess fat.

2. Add the remaining ingredients to slow cooker and mix well.

3. Cover and cook onlow for 6-8 hours

CALORIES	CARBS	SUGAR	FAT	PROTEIN	SODIUM
105	7.1	3.9	0.4	15.8	239
KCAL	GRAMS	GRAMS	GRAMS	GRAMS	MILLIGRAMS

HERB ROASTED CHICKEN WITH VEGETABLES

 SERVES **12**

 PREP TIME **20** **MINUTES**

 COOK TIME **8** **HOURS**

1. In a small bowl, mix paprika, thyme, salt and pepper. Rub them on the chicken breast evenly.

2. Place the onion and garlic in the slow cooker. Add chicken. Add the remaining vegetables around the chicken. Sprinkle vegetables with salt mixture. Drizzle with olive oil.

3. Cover and cook on low for 20 minutes

- **2 pounds** chicken tender
- **1/2 pound** beets, quartered
- **6** large Brussel sprouts, halved
- **4 cloves** garlic minced
- **1** medium onion, diced
- **1 tablespoon** olive oil
- **1 teaspoon** paprika
- **1 teaspoon** salt
- **1/2 teaspoon** dried thyme
- **1/2 teaspoon** ground black pepper

CALORIES	CARBS	SUGAR	FAT	PROTEIN	SODIUM
96	4.4	1.5	1.5	15.4	281
KCAL	GRAMS	GRAMS	GRAMS	GRAMS	MILLIGRAMS

JAMBALAYA CHICKEN AND SHRIMPS

 SERVES **12**

 PREP TIME **15** MINUTES

 COOK TIME **8.5** HOURS

- **1 pound** chicken tender, cut into 1-inch cubes

- **1 pound** shrimps, cooked, peeled and deveined

- **2** andouille sausages, sliced

- **1** 14.5-ounce **can** crushed tomatoes

- **2** green bell peppers, seeded and diced

- **1** medium onion, diced

- **1 cup** fat-free low sodium chicken broth

- **2 tablespoons** Cajun seasoning

- **1 teaspoon** hot sauce

1. Brown the meat. Transfer to slow cooker. Discard excess fat.

2. Add the remaining ingredients except shrimps to slow cooker and mix well.

3. Cover and cook on low for 6-8 hours. Add shrimps and cook on high for 30 minutes.

CALORIES	CARBS	SUGAR	FAT	PROTEIN	SODIUM
115	5.7	1.9	1.8	18.4	628
KCAL	GRAMS	GRAMS	GRAMS	GRAMS	MILLIGRAMS

HAM AND CAULIFLOWER STEW

SERVES
10

PREP TIME
5
MINUTES

COOK TIME
4
HOURS

1. Add all ingredients in the slow cooker.

2. Cover and cook on low for 4 hours.

- 1 pound extra lean ham, diced

- 1 pound cauliflower florets

- 3 cloves garlic, minced

- 2 cups fat-free low sodium chicken broth

- 1 cup shredded fat-free cheddar cheese

- 1/4 cup fat-free half-and-half

- 1/2 teaspoon onion powder

- 1/2 teaspoon salt

- 1/4 teaspoon ground black pepper

CALORIES	CARBS	SUGAR	FAT	PROTEIN	SODIUM
87	**5.5**	**1.4**	**1.4**	**13.0**	**648**
KCAL	GRAMS	GRAMS	GRAMS	GRAMS	MILLIGRAMS

CRUNCHY GERMAN SCHNITZEL CHOPS

 SERVES
8

 PREP TIME
15
MINUTES

 COOK TIME
6
HOURS

- **1 pound** 1-inch-thick butterfly pork chops, sliced lengthwise and pounded

- **1 egg white**, slightly beaten

- **1 cup** low-fat buttermilk

- **1 cup** whole wheat breadcrumbs

- **2 teaspoons** ground black pepper

- **1 teaspoon** garlic powder

- **1 teaspoon** paprika

- **1/2 teaspoon** salt

- Nonstick cooking spray

1. In a Medium bowl, combine egg white, buttermilk and all seasoning.

2. Apply cooking spray to the slow cooker.

3. Spray the Spread the bread crumbs on a plate. Dip the chops in the egg mixture then coat with breadcrumbs. Apply cooking spray to both sides of the pork chops before placing in the slow cooker.

4. Cover and cook on low for 6 hours

CALORIES	CARBS	SUGAR	FAT	PROTEIN	SODIUM
123	9.2	2.1	3.6	13.5	299
KCAL	GRAMS	GRAMS	GRAMS	GRAMS	MILLIGRAMS

PEPPER AND PORK CHOPS

 SERVES 8
 PREP TIME 5 **MINUTES**
 COOK TIME 8 **HOURS**

1. Place the pork chops in the slow cooker. Top with Green peppers and onion.

2. In a medium bowl, combine the remaining ingredients and pour over the vegetables.

3. Cover and cook on low 6-8 hours.

- 1 **pound** lean pork chops
- 1 8-ounce **can** tomato sauce
- 2 green bell peppers, sliced
- 1 medium onion, diced
- 2 **tablespoons** stevia
- 1 **tablespoon** apple cider vinegar
- 2 **teaspoons** Worcestershire sauce
- 1 **teaspoon** salt

CALORIES	CARBS	SUGAR	FAT	PROTEIN	SODIUM
92	6.9	2.4	2.4	12.4	567
KCAL	GRAMS	GRAMS	GRAMS	GRAMS	MILLIGRAMS

TERIYAKI PORK ROAST

SERVES
12

PREP TIME
10
MINUTES

COOK TIME
8
HOURS

- **2 pounds** pork roast
- **3/4 cup** unsweetened apple juice
- **2 tablespoons** low-sodium soy sauce
- **1 tablespoon** stevia
- **1 tablespoon** white vinegar
- **1 teaspoon** ground ginger
- **1/2 teaspoon** salt
- **1/4 teaspoon** garlic powder
- **1/4 teaspoon** pepper

1. Rub the salt onto the roast and place it in the slow cooker.

2. In a medium bowl, combine the remaining ingredients. Pour over the roast.

3. Cover and cook on low for 7-8 hours.

4. Slice the roast and serve with the sauce.

CALORIES	CARBS	SUGAR	FAT	PROTEIN	SODIUM
97	2.7	1.9	1.3	17.5	229
KCAL	GRAMS	GRAMS	GRAMS	GRAMS	MILLIGRAMS

ITALIAN PULL PORK

 SERVES
12

 PREP TIME
10
MINUTES

 COOK TIME
8
HOURS

1. Rub the salt, cayenne pepper and fennel seeds onto the roast and place it in the slow cooker. Top with onion and bell peppers.

2. Pour tomatoes over the roast.

3. Cover and cook on low for 6-8 hours.

4. Shred the meat and serve.

- **2 pounds** pork roast
- 1 14.5-ounce **can** diced tomatoes, with juice
- 1 medium onion, sliced
- 1 medium bell pepper, sliced
- **1 teaspoon** fennel seeds, crushed
- **1 teaspoon** salt
- **1/2 teaspoon** cayenne pepper

CALORIES	CARBS	SUGAR	FAT	PROTEIN	SODIUM
79	2.8	0.8	1.1	15.2	425
KCAL	GRAMS	GRAMS	GRAMS	GRAMS	MILLIGRAMS

COUNTRY STYLE PORK LOIN

SERVES
12

PREP TIME
10
MINUTES

COOK TIME
8
HOURS

- **2 pounds** pork roast

- **2 cups** fat-free low-sodium chicken broth

- **1 teaspoon** onion powder

- **1 teaspoon** dry mustard

- **1/2 teaspoon** salt

1. In a small bowl, combine onion powder, dry mustard and salt. Rub the mixture onto the pork roast and place it in the slow cooker.

2. Add broth. Cover and cook on low for 7-8 hours. Slice the roast and serve with juice.

CALORIES	CARBS	SUGAR	FAT	PROTEIN	SODIUM
69	0.3	0.0	1.0	15.0	301
KCAL	GRAMS	GRAMS	GRAMS	GRAMS	MILLIGRAMS

MEXICAN PULL PORK

 SERVES
16

 PREP TIME
15
MINUTES

 COOK TIME
6
HOURS

1. Rub the salt onto the roast and place it in the slow cooker. Top with green chilies and garlic.

2. In a medium bowl, combine the remaining ingredients. Pour over the roast.

3. Cover and cook on low for 6-8 hours. Shred the pork and serve.

- **2 pounds** pork roast, cut into 2-inch pieces
- **1** 4-ounce **can** diced green chilies
- **2 cloves** garlic, minced
- **1/2 cup** water
- **3 tablespoons** chipotle sauce
- **1/2 teaspoon** salt

CALORIES	CARBS	SUGAR	FAT	PROTEIN	SODIUM
71	0.8	0.1	1.0	14.8	351
KCAL	GRAMS	GRAMS	GRAMS	GRAMS	MILLIGRAMS

CRANBERRY APRICOT PORK ROAST

 SERVES **12**

 PREP TIME **10** MINUTES

 COOK TIME **9** HOURS

- **2 pounds** pork roast

- **2** shallots, finely chopped

- **1 cup** chopped cranberry

- **1/4 cup** dried apricots, chopped

- **1/4 cup** fresh orange juice

- **2 teaspoons** apple cider vinegar

- **1 teaspoon** dry mustard

- **1 teaspoon** grated fresh ginger

- **1 teaspoon** salt

1. Rub the salt onto the roast and place it in the slow cooker.

2. In a medium bowl, combine the remaining ingredients. Pour over the roast.

3. Cover and cook on slow for 7-9 hours.

4. Slice the roast and serve with the sauce.

CALORIES	CARBS	SUGAR	FAT	PROTEIN	SODIUM
82	3.7	2.4	1.1	14.9	384
KCAL	GRAMS	GRAMS	GRAMS	GRAMS	MILLIGRAMS

PORK CHILI

SERVES

12

PREP TIME

5

MINUTES

COOK TIME

10

HOURS

1. Add all ingredients except in the slow cooker. Stir to mix well.

2. Cover and cook on low for 8-10 hours. Shred the pork before serving.

- **1 1/2 pounds** pork tenderloin, cut into 2-inch pieces
- **1** 15-ounce **can** black beans, juice reserved
- **1** 16-ounce **jar** salsa
- **1** 4-ounce **can** diced green chilies
- **1** medium onion, chopped
- **1** red bell pepper, chopped
- **1/4 cup** fat free low sodium chicken broth
- **2 teaspoons** chili powder
- **1 teaspoon** dried oregano
- **1 teaspoon** ground cumin
- salt to taste

CALORIES	CARBS	SUGAR	FAT	PROTEIN	SODIUM
98	**11.0**	**1.5**	**1.3**	**14.0**	**634**
KCAL	GRAMS	GRAMS	GRAMS	GRAMS	MILLIGRAMS

PORK CARNITAS

 SERVES
12

 PREP TIME
5
MINUTES

 COOK TIME
10
HOURS

- **2 pounds** pork roast

- **2** bay leaves

- **1 tablespoons** chopped fresh thyme leaves

- **3/4 cup** fat-free low-sodium chicken broth

- **1 teaspoon** salt

- **1/2 teaspoon** ground black pepper

1. Rub the salt onto the roast and place it in the slow cooker.

2. Add the remaining ingredients on the side of the roast.

3. Cover and cook on low for 9-10 hours.

CALORIES	CARBS	SUGAR	FAT	PROTEIN	SODIUM
68	0.1	0.0	1.0	14.8	389
KCAL	GRAMS	GRAMS	GRAMS	GRAMS	MILLIGRAMS

TUSCAN PORK WITH FENNEL

 SERVES
8

 PREP TIME
10
MINUTES

 COOK TIME
10
HOURS

1. Place the fennel bulbs in the slow cooker

2. In a small bowl, mix together fennel seeds, rosemary, salt and pepper. Rub the seasoning on the pork and place in the slow cooker. Top with garlic.

3. In a medium bowl, combine broth and chicken base. Pour over.

4. Cover and cook on low for 8-10 hours

- **1 1/2 pounds** pork roast, cut into 4 slices
- **3 medium** fennel bulbs, diced
- **3 cloves** garlic, minced
- **3/4 cup** fat-free low sodium chicken broth
- **2 teaspoons** chicken base
- **2 teaspoons** fennel seeds
- **1 teaspoon** dried rosemary
- **1/2 teaspoon** salt
- **1/2 teaspoon** pepper

CALORIES	CARBS	SUGAR	FAT	PROTEIN	SODIUM
110	7.7	3.4	1.5	17.9	618
KCAL	GRAMS	GRAMS	GRAMS	GRAMS	MILLIGRAMS

MISO TOFU AND SHALLOTS

 SERVES
4

 PREP TIME
10
MINUTES

 COOK TIME
4
HOURS

- **1 pound** extra firm tofu, cut into 1/2-inch pieces

- **3** shallots, thinly sliced

- **1** green onion, finely chopped

- **2 tablespoons** miso paste

- **3 tablespoons** fat-free low-sodium chicken broth

- **1 teaspoon** olive oil

1. Place the shallot in the slow cooker. Line the tofu on top.

2. In a small bowl. Combine the remaining ingredients except green onion. Pour over tofu.

3. Cover and cook on low for 4 hours. Sprinkle with green onion and serve.

CALORIES	CARBS	SUGAR	FAT	PROTEIN	SODIUM
91	3.8	1.5	4.6	7.7	189
KCAL	GRAMS	GRAMS	GRAMS	GRAMS	MILLIGRAMS

VEGETABLES AND BEAN SOUP

 SERVES
16

 PREP TIME
10
MINUTES

 COOK TIME
9
HOURS

1. Add all ingredients in the slow cooker.

2. Cover and cook on low for 8-9 hours

- 2 15-ounce **cans** cannelloni beans, rinsed and drained
- 1 14.5-ounce **can** diced tomatoes
- 4 **stalks** celery, sliced
- 2 medium carrots, cut into 1-inch pieces
- 1 onion, diced
- 2 **cloves** garlic, minced
- 3 **cups** low sodium vegetable broth
- 1 bay leave
- 1/2 **teaspoon** crushed red pepper flakes
- salt and pepper to taste

CALORIES	CARBS	SUGAR	FAT	PROTEIN	SODIUM
60	12.1	1.6	0.0	3.6	198
KCAL	GRAMS	GRAMS	GRAMS	GRAMS	MILLIGRAMS

ZUCCHINI LASAGNA

 SERVES
16

 PREP TIME
30
MINUTES

 COOK TIME
9
HOURS

- **4** medium zucchini, sliced 1/8-inch thick

- **4 cups** tomato sauce

- **4 cups** fat-free shredded mozzarella cheese

- **8 ounces** fat-free ricotta cheese

- **1/4 cup** fat-free parmesan cheese

- **1** large egg

- **3/4 teaspoon** salt

- **1/4 teaspoon** ground black pepper

- Nonstick cooking Spray

1. Sprinkle zucchini with salt and let sit in a colander for about 30 minutes. Use paper towel to dry the slices

2. In a medium bowl combine egg, ricotta cheese and parmesan cheese. Set aside.

3. Spray the slow cooker. Spread 1 cup of tomato sauce evenly. Then cover with a layer of zucchini slices. Spread 1/4 of the egg mixture. Top with 1 cup of mozzarella cheese. Repeat the layers.

4. Cover and cook on low for 6-7 hours. Then turn the setting to warm and let it set for 1-2 hours before serving

CALORIES	CARBS	SUGAR	FAT	PROTEIN	SODIUM
89	9.0	4.0	0.4	12.3	762
KCAL	GRAMS	GRAMS	GRAMS	GRAMS	MILLIGRAMS

Cooking Information Summary

	Prep Time (min)	Cook time (hours)	No. of Ingredients	No. of condiments/ spice/herbs	Dairy Free?
Beef and Eggplant Casserole	10	5	4	4	N
Low Carb Pizza	15	6	7	1	N
Easy Swiss Steak	10	7	3	2	Y
Orange Beef	15	7	5	5	Y
Chinese Daikon Beef Stew	15	8	4	7	Y
Asian Braised Beef	20	8	6	6	Y
Traditional Texas Chili	20	8	7	5	Y
Riceless Cabbage Roll	30	8	6	4	N
Classic Beef Stew	10	8.5	5	3	Y
Shredded Beef Portobello Open Sandwich	15	8.5	2	7	Y
Broccoli and Beef	15	8.5	4	3	Y
Beef in Mushroom Sauce	25	8.5	4	2	Y
Round Roast in Apple and Onion Sauce	30	8.5	4	3	Y
Cuban Shredded Beef	30	10	5	2	Y
Spicy Beef Roast	15	10.5	3	2	Y
Buffalo Ranch Chicken	5	6	3	2	N
Creamy chicken with black beans	5	6	4	0	N
Creamy Mexican Chicken	5	6	4	1	N
Chicken Fajita Soup	5	6	6	3	Y
Vinegar Shredded Chicken	10	6	2	3	Y
BBQ Chicken	10	6	1	7	Y
Sweet and sour chicken	10	6	2	6	Y
Creamy Portobello Chicken	10	6	3	0	N
Chicken Cacciatore	15	6	6	2	Y

	Prep Time (min)	Cook Time (hours)	No. of ingredients	No. of Condiments/ spice/herbs	Dairy Free?
Creamy Lime Chicken	20	6	5	4	N
Chicken and Kale Soup	10	7	5	1	Y
White Chicken Chili	15	7	6	4	Y
Fiesta Chicken Soup	5	8	8	4	Y
Spinach Artichoke Chicken	5	8	8	0	N
Garlic Chicken Parmesan	10	8	3	5	N
Curry Chicken	10	8	4	5	Y
Mexican Turkey Casserole	10	8	7	3	N
Spicy Pepper Chicken	10	8	6	6	Y
Simple Turkey Chili	15	8	7	2	Y
Honey Mustard Chicken Stew	15	8	5	3	Y
Herb Roasted Chicken with Vegetables	20	8	5	2	Y
Jambalaya Chicken and Shrimps	15	8.5	7	2	Y
Ham and cauliflower stew	5	4	6	1	N
Crunchy German Schnitzel Chops	15	6	4	2	Y
Pepper and Pork Chops	5	8	4	3	Y
Teriyaki Pork Roast	10	8	2	5	Y
Italian Pull Pork	10	8	4	2	Y
Country Style pork loin	10	8	2	3	Y
Mexican Pull Pork	10	8	3	1	Y
Cranberry-Apricot Pork Roast	10	9	5	3	Y
Pork chili	5	10	7	3	Y
Pork Carnitas	5	10	2	2	Y
Tuscan Pork with Fennel	10	10	4	3	Y
Miso Tofu and Shallots	10	4	2	5	Y
Vegetable and Bean Soup	10	9	6	3	Y
Zucchini Lasagna	30	9	6	0	N

Nutrition Information Summary

	Calories (kCal)	Carbs (g)	Sugar (g)	Fat (g)	Protein (g)	Sodium (mg)
Beef and Eggplant Casserole	117	5.4	2.6	3.1	17.4	546
Low Carb Pizza	113	4.6	1.3	2.7	17.2	512
Easy Swiss Steak	108	7.0	2.4	3.0	13.3	307
Orange Beef	109	4.2	0.9	3.7	13.7	569
Chinese Daikon Beef Stew	107	3.3	1.6	2.8	17.4	218
Asian Braised Beef	114	4.3	1.8	2.9	17.1	248
Traditional Texas Chili	94	5.0	1.1	2.3	14.5	359
Riceless Cabbage Roll	111	6.1	3.4	3.7	14.2	360
Classic Beef Stew	113	5.3	1.2	2.7	17.3	291
Shredded Beef Portobello Open Sandwich	108	0.9	0.4	3.1	19.3	237
Broccoli and Beef	101	5.7	1.0	2.7	14.0	321
Beef in Mushroom Sauce	96	2.7	0.1	2.5	13.4	336
Round Roast in Apple and Onion Sauce	110	5.0	2.4	2.7	16.9	260
Cuban Shredded Beef	122	5.6	2.3	3.0	17.7	380
Spicy Beef Roast	102	2.7	0.6	2.7	16.8	217
Buffalo Ranch Chicken	109	0.3	0.1	3.4	17.4	481
Creamy chicken with black beans	116	10.1	2.7	0.8	16.8	562
Creamy Mexican Chicken	89	3.8	2.2	0.3	16.5	251
Chicken Fajita Soup	105	5.7	1.3	0.4	18.8	305
Vinegar Shredded Chicken	116	2.8	1.2	0.8	23.6	589
BBQ Chicken	98	2.9	1.8	2.6	14.7	273
Sweet and sour chicken	103	5.1	2.4	2.6	15.1	272
Creamy Portobello Chicken	116	7.2	1.4	1.4	17.5	663
Chicken Cacciatore	109	7.7	3.5	0.4	17.5	368

	Calories (kCal)	Carbs (g)	Sugar (g)	Fat (g)	Protein (g)	Sodium (mg)
Creamy Lime Chicken	91	2.5	0.6	1.7	15.4	209
Chicken and Kale Soup	95	3.9	0.6	0.5	18.1	125
White Chicken Chili	107	13.6	1.1	0.3	11.5	675
Fiesta Chicken Soup	98	11.0	1.6	0.7	12.1	299
Spinach Artichoke Chicken	123	11.0	3.5	0.3	17.3	586
Garlic Chicken Parmesan	99	4.4	0.0	1.5	16.1	437
Curry Chicken	125	6.5	1.7	3.0	17.1	387
Mexican Turkey Casserole	134	14.7	1.3	2.4	16.0	582
Spicy Pepper Chicken	94	3.7	1.3	1.4	16.3	161
Simple Turkey Chili	109	11.5	3.2	0.8	14.9	397
Honey Mustard Chicken Stew	105	7.1	3.9	0.4	15.8	239
Herb Roasted Chicken with Vegetables	96	4.4	1.5	1.5	15.4	281
Jambalaya Chicken and Shrimps	115	5.7	1.9	1.8	18.4	628
Ham and cauliflower stew	87	5.5	1.4	1.4	13.0	648
Crunchy German Schnitzel Chops	123	9.2	2.1	3.6	13.5	299
Pepper and Pork Chops	92	6.9	2.4	2.4	12.4	567
Teriyaki Pork Roast	97	2.7	1.9	1.3	17.5	229
Italian Pull Pork	79	2.8	0.8	1.1	15.2	425
Country Style pork loin	69	0.3	0.0	1.0	15.0	301
Mexican Pull Pork	71	0.8	0.1	1.0	14.8	351
Cranberry-Apricot Pork Roast	82	3.7	2.4	1.1	14.9	384
Pork chili	98	11.0	1.5	1.3	14.0	634
Pork Carnitas	68	0.1	0.0	1.0	14.8	389
Tuscan Pork with Fennel	110	7.7	3.4	1.5	17.9	618
Miso Tofu and Shallots	91	3.8	1.5	4.6	7.7	189
Vegetable and Bean Soup	60	12.1	1.6	0.0	3.6	198
Zucchini Lasagna	89	9.0	4.0	0.4	12.3	762

THANK YOU FOR READING!

After your bariatric surgery, what you eat play a significant role in healing and nourishing your body.

I hope this book has provide you some new inspiration. Thank you again for picking up my book and going through it.

STELLA LAYNE 2017